**INFORMATION HANDLING
PRACTICE:** Challenges for 1

INFORMATION HANDLING IN GENERAL
PRACTICE: CHALLENGES FOR THE FUTURE

Edited by
R. H. WESTCOTT and R. V. H. JONES

CROOM HELM
London & Sydney

© 1988 R. H. Westcott and R. V. H. Jones
Croom Helm Ltd, 11 New Fetter Lane,
London EC4P 4EE
Croom Helm Australia, 44–50 Waterloo Road,
North Ryde, 2113, New South Wales

British Library Cataloguing in Publication Data

Information handling in general practice:
challenges for the future.
1. Family medicine — Information services — Management
I. Westcott, R.H. II. Jones, R.V.H.
362.1'72   R729.5.G4
ISBN 0-7099-5228-7

Printed in Great Britain by
St. Edmundsbury Press Ltd
Bury St. Edmunds, Suffolk

Contents

Preface	vii
Acknowledgements	viii
Introduction	ix
Contributors	xi

Part One: Past History: Information in Perspective	1
1. Medical Records in the Practice *Ian Tait*	3
2. Information for Practice Management: A Historical Review *Mike Pringle*	16
3. The Literature of General Practice *Simon Barley*	25
4. Information for Patients *Susan Clayton*	40
5. A Review of Information for People *Richard Westcott*	50

Part Two: Present: Information Needs	59
6. Information for Doctors *Brian Higginson*	61
7. Information for People *Joan Mant and Richard Westcott*	79

Part Three: What Technology Offers Now	87
8. What Microcomputers Offer Doctors Now *Stewart Reid and Bob Jones*	89
9. What Computers and Broadcasting Offer Patients *John Chisholm*	104

Part Four: In the Pipeline	119
10. Clinical Information and Data Bases *Ellie Scrivens and Claudine Hornyold-Strickland*	121
11. Aids to Diagnosis — an Impertinent Look at some Pertinent Questions *Tim de Dombal*	129
12. Aids to Clinical Management *Bob Jones*	149
13. Artificial Intelligence *John Fox, Andrzej Glowinski and Michael O'Neil*	157
14. Electronic Technology and Practice Management *Mike Pringle*	180
15. Health Information for Patients *Neil Carson and Peter MacIsaac*	197
16. Information Technology and Public Health Education *Alan Maryon-Davis*	212

Part Five: Challenges for the Future   221
17. Computers in General Practice — the Future
    David Metcalfe   223
18. The Health Care Paradox — Implications for Computing in Primary Health Care   *Nigel Stott*   231
19. Why Computerised Clinical Records are Indispensable   *Bob Johnson*   238
20. General Practice at the Crossroads   *Mike Fitter and Bob Garber*   253
21. The Final Account   *Richard Turner*   270

Conclusion: The Way Ahead   *Bob Jones and Richard Westcott*   284

Index   286

Preface

Attitudes towards information about health and illness are changing. Articles in magazines and newspapers, programmes on radio and television are evidence of a steadily increasing interest in health matters among the general public. Patients demand to know more. Attitudes are also changing among general practitioners who are becoming aware of the needs of patients to know more about their illnesses and treatment, to be involved in choice.

At the same time electronic innovations capable of transforming the amount of information which is available are about to burst into daily life — in homes, in schools, in hospitals, in surgeries.

In our view this combination of circumstances is likely to have a fundamental effect on the practice of medicine in the community. We have asked 22 individual authors to provide a historical perspective to the scene as it is today, and to look into the future. We hope that general practitioners and a wider audience will find the text stimulating and provocative.

Finally, while the historical review contained in the opening chapters is largely based on events in Britain, the remainder of the book draws on experience in America, in New Zealand and Australia as well as in the UK. We believe that the questions posed are, or will become, relevant wherever microcomputers are used as tools in general practice.

RICHARD WESTCOTT
ROBERT JONES

Acknowledgements

We should like to express a debt of gratitude to our authors who have cheerfully accepted editorial suggestions and pruning in the interest of consistency. We trust that our combined efforts have minimised the disadvantages of multiple authorship without blurring their distinctive voices.

Among individuals who have provided advice and helpful criticism we are particularly grateful to Dr Peter Pritchard and to Professor Clem McDonald of Indianapolis, USA.

Heather Hutchinson deserves our special thanks for combining her secretarial duties with quietly compensating for our deficiencies.

Introduction

The subject of health information and the way it is handled is a large one. At first sight the list of contents on page v may appear disorganised and confusing. The purpose of this introduction is to explain the structure on which the text is based, so that readers can follow through individual themes more easily and can understand their relationship to the book as a whole.

Part 1: in order to appreciate the nature and speed of change it is necessary to know how the present position has been reached. In this part five chapters present an historical review of the information about health and illness which has become available to general practitioners, to patients and to the general public from the early nineteenth century to the present day.

Part 2: the information needs of patients, the general public and of family practitioners as they are currently perceived are summarised in this section.

Part 3 describes what computers at this moment can offer patients and doctors. It reviews the extent to which their information needs are being met by electronic technology.

In *Part 4* we move into the future. In a series of chapters whose subject-matter broadly corresponds to the chapters in *Part One*, developments which are now in the pipeline and are expected to be in service use within a few years are described.

In *Part 5*, the final part, a general practitioner, a community physician, a psychologist and two professors of general practice present their personal views as to the challenges which the profession will face if, as expected, electronic technology becomes all-pervasive.

The editors append a short conclusion.

Contributors

Simon Barley MB FRCGP
General Practitioner, Sheffield, UK

Neil E. Carson MB BS FRACGP FRACP
Professor and Head of Department of Community Medicine, Monash University, Victoria, Australia

John W. Chisholm BA MB BChir MRCGP DRCOG
General Practitioner, Twyford, UK
Chairman, Practice Organisation Sub-committee, General Medical Services Committee

Susan Clayton BA MA
Lecturer in Social Policy, University of Lancaster, UK

F. T. de Dombal MD FRCS
Reader in Clinical Information Sciences, St James University Hospital, Leeds, UK

Michael J. Fitter BSc PhD
Senior Research Fellow, MRC/ESRC Social and Applied Psychology Unit, University of Sheffield, UK

John Fox BSc PhD
Head of Biomedical Computing Unit, Imperial Cancer Research Fund, London, UK

J. Robert Garber BSc MSc
Management Consultant and MRC/ESRC Psychology Unit, University of Sheffield, UK

Andrzej Glowinski MA BM BCh
Clinical Fellow, Imperial Cancer Research Fund, London, UK

Brian M. Higginson MB BS DRCOG DO
General Practitioner, Hastings, UK

Claudine Hornyold-Strickland MBA Insead
PhD Student, London Business School, UK

Robert A. Johnson MA MRCGP MRCP(Psych) PhD
General Practitioner, Greater Manchester, UK
Member of British Computer Society

Robert V. H. Jones MA FRCGP
General Practitioner, Seaton, Devon, UK
Honorary Senior Lecturer, Department of General Practice, University of Exeter, UK

Joan Mant BA
Vice President, National Association for Patient Participation, UK

Peter MacIsaac MB BS
General Practitioner, Camperdown, Victoria, Australia
Lecturer, Department of Community Medicine, Monash University, Victoria, Australia

Alan Maryon-Davis MSc MRCP FFCM
Senior Medical Advisor and Director of the Health Division, Health Education Authority, UK

David H. H. Metcalfe FRCGP MFCM
Professor of General Practice, University of Manchester, UK

Michael O'Neil BSc MRCP
Clinical Fellow, Imperial Cancer Research Fund, London, UK

Michael A. L. Pringle MD DRCOG MRCGP
General Practitioner, Collingham, Newark, UK
Senior Lecturer in General Practice, University of Nottingham, UK

J. Stewart Reid MB ChB MRCGP MRNZCGP
General Practitioner, Lower Hutt, New Zealand
Clinical Lecturer, Wellington Clinical School, New Zealand

Ellie Scrivens PhD
Lecturer in Public Sector Management, The London Business School, UK

Nigel C. H. Stott BSc FRCP FRCGP
Professor, Department of General Practice, University of Wales College of Medicine, UK

Ian G. Tait MA DCH FRCGP
General Practitioner, Aldeburgh, UK

Richard D. Turner MB ChB MFCM
Specialist in Community Medicine, Yorkshire Regional Health Authority, UK

Richard H. Westcott MA MRCGP DRCOG DCH
General Practitioner, South Molton, North Devon, UK

Part 1

Past History: Information in Perspective

1

Medical Records in the Practice

Ian Tait

THE HISTORY OF THE CLINICAL RECORD IN BRITISH GENERAL PRACTICE

The general practitioner emerged in the early part of the nineteenth century as the major provider of medical care for the population of Britain. The records that he kept were very simple. They were generally confined to his 'Day Book' in which would be recorded the names of patients seen or visited, the drugs given and the fees charged. A minimum of clinical detail was included. The rest lay buried in the doctor's head, or disappeared.

EARLY HISTORY

The first significant attempt to influence the clinical record-keeping habits of general practitioners came with the Lloyd George National Insurance Act of 1911. Under this Act, general practitioners were to provide general medical services for insured male patients and to receive a capitation fee for each person registered on their list. This was a time when there was some anxiety about the health of the working population of Britain. Facts were needed: the potential value of the statistical information available as the result of the medical care given under the terms of the Act was recognised by the Government, and general practitioners participating in the scheme were asked to 'keep such medical records as might be required of them under their conditions of service'.

The records they were required to keep consisted of cards recording cases seen with their diagnoses. These cards were returned for central analysis at the end of each year. They were thus of little use in the continuing clinical care of patients. Perhaps the most significant aspect of this first attempt to introduce records into general practice was quite incidental; namely that doctors were supplied with metal boxes in which to keep the record cards.

During the 1914–18 War general practitioners were relieved of the requirement to keep records. After the War an important committee was set up (The Rolleston Committee).[1] Its task was to advise the Government as to what kind of records GPs should be required to keep under the terms of the Insurance Act. In their conclusions the Committee made a very clear and important statement to the effect that the primary purpose of the record should be to improve the quality of patient care, 'that is to say, the ways in which the keeping of records may contribute to the more efficient treatment of patients, both by the doctor who makes the record and by the doctors under whose care the same patient may come in subsequent illnesses'.

Two important principles for general practice records are expressed or implied in this statement. Firstly that the quality of the medical record itself has a significant influence on the quality of medical care that a doctor is likely to provide, and secondly, that the record has a function to perform in ensuring effective continuity of medical care when a patient is to be treated by a number of different doctors at different times.

Having defined the objective of the clinical record with admirable clarity the Committee found it much more difficult to translate this into definite recommendations about the design and content of the record. They were, however, unanimous over one thing: that was that the size of the records should be such that they could be stored in the tin boxes already supplied to general practitioners! It is indeed ironic to think that our present struggles with our record envelopes are the result of tin boxes supplied to GPs in the early part of this century for records that had quite a different purpose. Nevertheless, much credit goes to the Rolleston Committee. It defined the essential clinical function of our records, and succeeded in introducing a uniform system of record-keeping into general practice.

The form of the record they advised was adequate to meet the relatively simple demands made upon it at the time. When the National Health Service was introduced in 1948, this record was accepted virtually unaltered as the system to be used throughout British general practice.

The early years of the Health Service were hard times. General practitioners were ill-prepared and ill-supported for the formidable tasks that confronted them. This was also true of the medical record. The Collings Report (1950), which was based on a personal review of a wide range of general practices, revealed a state of affairs which seemed depressing in the extreme.[2] Collings remarks that during his visits he never saw anything approaching good records. However, even in those early days there were those who recognised the importance of the clinical records for good practice, and sought for ways to improve them.

Stephen Taylor, in his influential book *Good general practice*,[3] which was based on his own extensive study of general practitioners at work, wrote:

> One has reached the conclusion that the key to good general practice is the keeping of good clinical records. Time and again one has seen a quick glance through a well kept record card provide either a diagnosis or an essential point of treatment.

The foundation of the College of General Practitioners in 1953 provided a focus for reformers interested in better records. One of these was Dr Walford of Felstead, who, as early as 1955, writing in the *College Newsletter*, had some very practical suggestions for improving records which we are still some way from achieving on a general scale today.

> It is suggested that a special continuation card of a distinctive colour — a Summary Continuation Card — should be used to convey the patient's history from one doctor to the next. On this Summary Card should be entered important illnesses, laboratory reports and certain personal details that have a profound effect on the medical life of the patient. Exactly what constitutes an 'important illness' in this context is rather difficult to define. Perhaps it is 'a disease whose absence from the Summary Card would materially handicap a subsequent practitioner, or delay his arrival at a diagnosis'.[4]

It would be difficult to improve on that description of an effective Summary Card.

THE A4 DEBATE

By the late 1960s the major problem for the record seemed to many people to be the inability of the record envelope to store records and reports in a way that made them easily accessible. In 1965 the Tonbridge Report had recommended standard A4 size records for hospitals and local health authorities. The idea that general practice should also have A4 records began to gain attention.

In 1967 Dr Loudon and his colleagues in Wantage gained support for a project for the trial of A4 records in two local practices. The results of this study were reported in 1971,[5] and appeared to show that A4 records would be welcomed in general practice. In the same year the Annual Conference of representatives of LMCs passed an important resolution, which is worth quoting:

> That as a matter of policy future medical records should be of a size to contain unfolded paper of A4 size and should be made available to those doctors who wish to use it provided that a firm undertaking is given by the Department of Health to finance all consequent alterations to equipment and premises arising therefrom. (*British Medical Journal*, 1971, *3* (7), 71)

The qualifying conditions should be noted. This resolution committed the GMSC to negotiate with the Government for a change to a total A4 record system for general practice, but at the same time to get it paid for, whatever the cost. A Joint Working Party was set up which designed an A4 record system for general practice. This even got so far as to be offered to any general practitioner who wished to adopt it. But protracted negotiations failed to resolve the thorny question of who should pay the cost of providing the equipment and space needed for the records. In Scotland things were better managed, and today practices are provided with A4 records. In England and Wales the long argument over cost led to stalemate and, finally, to the withdrawal by the DHSS of the offer to provide A4 records except to those practices who had already introduced them, a result that does indeed seem to be the worst of both worlds.

The A4 debate had now, in many people's view, been overtaken by the question of the computerisation of records in general practice. Whether this is true or not, the content of the record and its organisation remains a matter of central importance, and it is to this theme that we must return.

ORGANISING THE CONTENT OF THE RECORD

The first serious study of the content of general practice records was carried out by Cormack in his MD thesis of 1970.[6] In this and subsequent reports Cormack exposed serious deficiencies of all kinds of important information in the records of patients in general practice. In seeking reasons for this he identified the two major faults of the record as firstly the absence of space for recording important background information set aside from day-to-day recordings, and, secondly, the fact that letters have to be folded, often more than once, to fit the record envelope. He wrote:

> Much thought needs to be directed towards the provision of space clearly set aside for the recording of background information of a permanently valuable nature, easily accessible and separate from those items of day-to-day recording of more ephemeral interest.

The story of general practice records since that time has really been one of slow recognition of the truth of this statement. The general practitioner needs a defined range of information for the optimum care of his patients. This information requires to be collected and recorded, and the structure of the record must facilitate both its recording and its recall.

With the failure of efforts to introduce an A4 record system on any general basis, many of those interested in record reform in general practice began to concentrate on defining the range of information needed, and in designing structured cards for its storage and retrieval which were compatible with the existing record system.

PROBLEM-ORIENTATED MEDICAL RECORDS

In the early 1970s there was considerable interest in problem-orientated records. This arose from the work of Lawrence Weed in America. His writings, and still more his charismatic performances on his visit to Britain, won him influential converts amongst record reformers in general practice. Although the pure problem-orientated record is hardly a practical instrument for British general practice, certain principles enunciated by Weed were very influential in guiding the thinking of those who were attempting to improve our present record.[7]

First, the idea of a defined data base. Weed pointed out that every branch of medicine needs to define the range of information it requires in order to carry out its professional task, and that this was as true in general practice as in other specialties. He challenged us to declare what information we should have about patients on our medical lists, and then to take steps to collect it and record it appropriately so that it could be used.

Second, he pointed out that doctors deal with problems more than with established diagnoses, and that what the doctor needs to be reminded of are the problems he has to attend to that are unsolved, i.e. those that are still 'active' problems. Weed suggested the use of a problem list which would contain problems expressed at the doctor's honest level of understanding. These might be physical, psychological or social. They might be well-defined or ill-defined, but if ill-defined the problem should be thus expressed: e.g. 'chest pain' not 'Fibrositis', or 'angina', if the diagnosis was still uncertain.

Third, Weed defined a system for continuation notes which was designed to make explicit the reasons for the doctor's conclusions and actions. Weed called this 'The logic pathway of the doctor's problem solving'. His system would help doctors understand subsequently why things had been done, as well as what was done. Such an idea has obvious relevance for medical care in general practice, particularly where more than one doctor is involved. Furthermore it has great relevance for medical education because it is only by being able to assess how a doctor sets about solving clinical problems that we can help him to improve that essential skill.

His system suggests that follow-up notes should have the following structure:[8]

S Subject information — what the patient reports.
O Objective information — what the doctor finds.
A Assessment — what the doctor thinks.
P Plan — what the doctor decides to do (on the basis of his assessment)

    Dx diagnostic plans
    Rx treatment and management plans
    Ed education plans — includes a record of important statements made to the patient.

All these concepts seemed attractive and relevant to general practice records, and in one way or another many of them have been incorporated into suggestions for reform of our records.

TOWARDS THE COMPUTER AGE

This history of general practice records in the past ten years has been much influenced by the potential contribution that computers might make. In the early days there was a tendency to think of them as some kind of magic answer that would do the job without anyone having to take much thought. The first discovery made by any doctor who became involved in computerisation of his records was that he needed to structure and organise his existing records, and the information in them, before he could get that information into computerised form.

IMPROVING THE EXISTING RECORD

The use of structured cards of various kinds to organise information in general practice records has been a feature of the past ten years. Tait, in 1974, designed a series of background data cards and carried out a pilot study of their use in general practice with the help of the Cardew Stanning Foundation. These cards subsequently became available for general practice through the RCGP Central Information Centre. Many doctors developed variations of these cards for their own use. Indeed, a feature of general practice records in recent years has been the rich variety of 'improved records' that individual GPs have devised. They include cards compatible with the FPC record envelope, A4 records and computerised record systems.

But one of the great advantages of the record system in British general practice is its basic uniformity. It is important to try to preserve this uniformity. The record is personal to the patient and moves from doctor to doctor with the patient. As a record of an individual's health history throughout his life it has a huge potential, which has been quite unrealised. The arrival of computers in general practice should make this a great deal easier, but it will not be so unless we preserve some standard structure. The problem at the present time is that getting agreement over reform is so difficult. Somehow we must capitalise on individual initiatives, improve our records and at the same time preserve a common format for them.

GOOD RECORDS FOR ALL

What I have so far described is the story of our efforts to improve our records in general practice from the simple envelope and card introduced by the Rolleston Committee in 1920. It has been largely the story of individual reformers. But what really matters is not what the individual does, but what is done by the generality of doctors. No story of records in general practice would be complete without some mention of the way in which the records in teaching practices have been improved by the simple expedient of requiring improvement before approval can be granted. Practices which have been persuaded in this way to improve their records are always delighted that it has happened. If we are really to improve our records it does seem that we need carrots, and sometimes even sticks! The situation at the present time is that the Joint Committee for Postgraduate Training (the body that sets standards for teaching practices), has required that records in teaching practices should reach certain minimum standards. They should have letters and cards fixed in date order; should have a completed Summary Card and a Drug Card that is accurate, with up-to-date information on drugs being given and dosage. The continuation notes should be legible and make it easy to identify active problems in some way. This requirement has resulted in a very marked improvement in the general standard of records in teaching practices. It may seem extraordinary that such minimum standards are not already universal in general practice; sadly they are not. What the requirements of the JCPT have shown, however, is that given a little extra motivation a significant improvement in the standard of records in general practice can be achieved.

GETTING OUR PRESENT RECORDS STRAIGHT — THE CHALLENGE OF TODAY

This story of our records in general practice has now reached the present time, and must begin to look to the future. The arrival of the computer age has presented all of us in general practice with a challenge to which we simply have to respond. But as we have seen, before we can do so properly we have to get our present record system into order. This is not an optional extra but an essential preliminary. Much work is currently taking place in this area, and there is now general agreement about the essential steps we have to take.

The most important of these is to decide on the range of information we wish to record (the data base). An example of such a data base is given below:

P Past history: to include relevant facts and risk factors in the medical, family and social history. In considering how much detail is needed we can do no better than remember Walford's definition. We should include any fact 'whose absence would materially handicap a practitioner or delay his arrival at a diagnosis'.
A Active problems: some way is needed of keeping before the practitioner's attention all the active problems he needs to attend to. In manual records this is most conveniently done by some form of highlighting in the continuation notes.
R Report and letters: relevant reports and letters need to be easily available. The volume of these increases all the time in today's general practice. In some chronic cases only the use of an A4 file will cope with the bulk of letters and reports. In all cases it is essential that they are fixed in date order.
T Treatment: the problem of knowing for certain what drugs a patient is taking, and in what dosage, is always with us, particularly in long-term care, where changes of treatment and dosages are common. Special arrangements require to be made in the record to cope with this.
S Sensitivity: this may be to drugs or other agents. Sensitivities need to be recorded in a way that ensures that they are noticed.

For those addicted to acronyms, these are the PARTS of an adequate data base for general practice.[9]

Once we have defined our data base we can set about deciding how we collect and store the information we need.

Many practices are developing some form of questionnaire which can be completed by the patient, and which can provide much of the background information needed. Such a questionnaire can be reviewed in an initial interview when the patient joins the practice, at which time points can be clarified, and additional information obtained.

There is a real problem of knowing how to store information in our existing records. We cannot really do this without the use of some additional structured card that, in Cormack's words, 'provides a space, clearly set aside for the recording of background information of a permanently valuable nature'.

The minimum requirements are as follows:

(1) Summary Card. This needs to include not only medical events but significant facts from the family and social history.

(2) Treatment or Drug Card, which acts as an index to drugs given, and should include a section for recording sensitivities.

(3) Flow Sheet for the recording of long-term treatment in chronic cases where drugs and dosages change.

(4) Some form of Repeat Prescription Card carried by the patient and presented when drugs are needed. This card should indicate how often prescriptions have been given and when the patient should next see the doctor.

Advances in information technology will doubtless alter the form in which this material is recorded, but not its substance.

RECORDS FOR SHARED CARE

A new and welcome feature in general practice is the development of arrangements or protocols for shared care of patients with hospital departments. Such a system has been in existence for antenatal care for many years but it is now more common to find it extended to conditions such as diabetes and hypertension. Specifically designed record cards that facilitate the sharing of information between the hospital and general practice have been developed in all these areas. Once again computers may greatly simplify this process in the future, but we will all benefit if we have sorted out our ideas 'on paper' first.

A MEDICAL RECORD FOR THE PATIENT

Recently there has been a movement for the patient to be more actively involved as a 'partner' in the decisions involved in his medical care. This tendency has been paralleled by a recognition that the patient can, and perhaps should, be encouraged to take a greater responsibility for the quality and use of his own medical record.

Once again we may note that this has already been happening in a quiet way with the co-operation cards commonly used in antenatal care and in diabetic clinics. We may expect to see an extension of this idea in the future, so that the patient carries with him a general record of his health care.

The Royal Australian College of General Practitioners has designed a personal health record card which is carried by the patient, and similar records are used in France. British general practice will need to develop its own patient-held record. Once again we must hope this will be of uniform design.

CONFIDENTIALITY AND THE MEDICAL RECORD

Several factors are making the confidentiality of the medical record an issue of growing importance. Firstly there is the computerisation of information, which makes it potentially available to anyone who can gain access to the data base, perhaps even illegally. Secondly, the increase in number of professionals and other paramedical personnel working in general practice, and having legitimate, or sometimes illegitimate, access to patient records. Thirdly, the greatly increased amount of information which is now to be found in patients' records, some of it of a highly confidential nature. We also need to note that a much more articulate and potentially critical point of view is being expressed by patient associations and other consumer organisations. This tendency will almost certainly increase.

We in general practice need to develop clear policies for protecting the confidentiality of patients' records, and to make those policies absolutely explicit to ourselves, our staff and our patients.

RECORDS AND THE PRACTICE POPULATION

We in general practice are first and foremost personal doctors but, increasingly, we are being asked to recognise that we have a responsibility to our patients when they are healthy, not only when they are ill. We thus have a concern for our practice population as a whole, particularly in relation to preventive medicine and health education. A practice needs record systems to support these activities. Often the existing medical record can act in this way, for instance by recording smoking or dietary or drinking habits, or weight and blood pressure over time. In so far as this is true it is part of the developing history of the clinical record in general practice.

In some areas of work, however, other forms of record system such as age/sex registers and disease indices are needed. Such additions to our traditional clinical record will be considered later in this book.

THE FUTURE

In terms of the long history of medicine the history of general practice is short. The history, if we can call it that, of an appropriate record system for general practice is very short indeed.

Instead of feeling that everything has already been decided, and is somehow unalterable, we should see ourselves as pioneers in a new and exciting period of development of the record in and for general practice. In achieving high standards and new roles in the care of our patients we will find appropriate records will be second only in importance to that magic complex of knowledge, experience and personal qualities that constitutes the 'good doctor'. I am almost tempted to say equal first, because I no longer believe it will be possible, in the general practice of the future, to be a good doctor without good records.

REFERENCES

1. Rolleston, Sir Humphrey (1920) *Report of the Interdepartmental Committee on Insurance Medical Records.* HMSO, London
2. Collings, J. (1950) General practice in England today: a reconnaisance. *Lancet, 1,* 555–85
3. Taylor, S. (1954) *Good general practice.* Oxford University Press, London
4. Walford, P.A. (1955) General practice records. *College of General Practitioners Newsletter, 7,* 53
5. Loudon, I.S.L. (1971) Hawkey, Loudon and Greenhaigh and Bungay. New record folder for use in general practice. *British Medical Journal, 4,* 667
6. Cormack, J.J.C. (1970) The medical record envelope — a case for reform. *Royal College of General Practitioners, 20,* 333
7. Weed, L. (1969) Medical records that guide and teach. *New England Journal of Medicine, 278,* 593–600 and 652–7
8. Tait, I.G. (1977) The clinical record in British general practice. *British Medical Journal, 2,* 683–8

9. Tait, I. and Follis, P. (1980) *Is this a record — improving records in general practice.* Schering Educational Services, Burgess Hill, Sussex

2

Information for Practice Management: A Historical Review

Mike Pringle

INTRODUCTION

In the twentieth century general practice has moved from an almost total reliance on an individual doctor's memory to the possibility of highly structured record-keeping. On the coat-tails of this change has come an awareness of the role of practice management. While this is personified by the introduction of practice managers it is illustrated more tangibly by the arrival of practice card index registers and computers, by the production of books [1,2] and the holding of courses about practice management.

This chapter reviews the major changes in the structure of general practice that have catalysed these developments in practice management, and the ways that information systems have evolved. Through a discussion of the past and present sources of practice information, the assets and drawbacks of currently available internal, external and community statistics relating to practices and their environments are explored.

THE HISTORICAL PERSPECTIVE

While the patient's medical record can be traced back to case histories inscribed on the columns of the temple ruins at Epidaurus, near Athens, in 1134 BC, the first recorded attempt at derived statistics occurred in 1622. At this time Captain John Graunt analysed the 'Bills of Mortality' and found that, in common with today, mortality rates were higher in urban areas than in the country.[3]

While such epidemiological studies became commoner they did

not rely substantially on the records in general practice, which were still rudimentary at the start of this century. In 1912 the first of three major revolutions occurred. The National Health Insurance Scheme covered all workers who earned less than £160 per year for the cost of general practitioner care and medicines, in addition to unemployment and sickness benefit. From this was derived one of the most crucial features of modern general practice, namely patient registration with a doctor. This principle was reinforced by the subsequent widespread introduction of 'sick clubs' in which a doctor undertook primary care for a few pence a week.

The second major event for both the profession and practice management occurred with the formation of the National Health Service in 1948. This extended patient registration with a general practitioner of choice to every person in the country, and the doctor was paid a capitation fee. This had the effects of extending free primary care to all, and extending patient registration and identification. However, the system of capitation acted as a disincentive for doctors to develop their services: the less they invested in their services, the more they had left over as income.[4]

The gauntlet of responsibility for a defined patient group was not taken up until the 'General Practice Charter' in 1965. In a wide-ranging review and reformation of the financial structure of general practice, the pattern of the past 20 years was defined. By instituting reimbursements for premises and staff the scope for practice development without detriment to the doctors was increased, and items of service payments recognised the fact that financial incentives were the most likely stimulation of preventive care. Extra payments for group practice and doctors working in under-resourced areas changed the face of general practice. In 1952, 43 per cent of doctors were single-handed, but by 1980 the proportion had fallen to 14 per cent.

The increasing complexity of medical practice, and the advent of group practices, meant that practice management in the second half of this century could no longer be entrusted to the memory of a single doctor. The need for tools for practice management, and the generation of statistics, became increasingly apparent. While the introduction of the NHS had stimulated the widespread introduction of written medical record envelopes to general practice, the charter was followed by interest in the contents of these records. The resultant improved recording of medical information acted as a stimulus for the development of practice management tools.

These can be considered under the broad headings of internal registers (such as patient-based age–sex or disease registers), internal practice information (spasmodic or continuous audit of workload and practice activities), and external practice information. This latter includes information about practice activity gathered by outside agencies, statistics relating to other medical services and data on the community served. Each of these three areas will be examined in turn.

INTERNAL REGISTERS

In a review[5] credit is given for the earliest introduction of an age–sex register to Dr C. A. K. Watts in 1960. Concurrently ideas for a card index disease register[6] and a practice index[7-9] were developing. From others came the concepts of a diagnostic index (E book) and card index age–sex registers using RCGP standard format cards.

By 1971, 320 practices were using the RCGP age–sex cards both for defining the demography of the practice and, in half the cases, for preventive care recalling. By 1977 the number of practices with age–sex registers had risen to 850, and in 1985 a survey in the West Midlands found that 52 per cent of practices had registers.[10] The reported uses varied from screening and surveillance, to disease recording and research. As in previous reports these age–sex registers were being used for setting up health education programmes, although the extent to which this occurred was not reported. While the accuracy of age–sex registers has been widely doubted[11,12] their use as a basis for other practice registers appears widespread.

It must, however, be observed that many practices have installed age–sex registers primarily in order to meet the criteria for trainers in vocational training schemes. It appears anecdotally that many age–sex registers are under-used and under-maintained, and that they are the subject of more wishful thinking than hard practice.

As early as 1963 the problems with diagnostic labels in general practice were acknowledged,[8] and from this evolved the RCGP classification of disease.[13] Later the International Classification of Health Problems of Primary Care[14] was developed and updated.[15] At first notes were colour-coded, or patients recorded in E-books. Later the age–sex cards themselves were used to code these patients with selected important diagnoses.[16] More recently computer systems have been used both to hold the age–sex registers and to link them to preventive care files and disease indices.

Interest in repeat prescribing only began after the formation of the NHS, when the new prescriptions did not include the previous possibility of instructing the chemist to repeat the medication.[17] Early attempts to control such prescriptions involved patient-held cards[18] but separate repeat prescribing sheets in the notes were also used. The advent of the general practice computer has radically changed the way in which practice registers are perceived and used, and the organization of repeat prescribing. The present position is summarized in Chapter 8.

The evaluation of the 150 practices involved in the 'Micros for GPs' scheme, however, reported that for repeat prescribing 'in some practices a little time was saved by using the computer; in others it took longer. Time reductions were generally offset by the necessary housekeeping and updating activities associated with the computer system'.[19] Computerised recall systems have been shown to increase practice income and preventive care uptake,[20] but so have manual systems. It appears that current general practice computers are equal to manual registers in efficiency but have advantages in speed and flexibility. Against this must be placed the cost and workload involved.

INTERNAL PRACTICE INFORMATION

The advent of the GP Charter had two important repercussions for internal practice information — the formation of group practices and the payments for items of preventive service. In the pre-Charter days the need for a doctor to generate statistics was limited to consultation rates, but since 1965 there have been practical and financial reasons for practices to generate internal data. In the larger group practices up to 25,000 patients may be registered, of whom 3750 will be women aged 35–55 suitable for cervical cytology call and recall, and 1750 children under five for immunisation and developmental screening.[21] To maximise practice income not only must these patients be identified and followed up, but also the practice needs to offer patients tetanus immunisation and ensure that claims are made for all women receiving contraceptive advice. This notional practice will have 14,000 adults aged between 30 and 70 who require blood pressure surveillance.

Some practices approached this problem by setting up registers — usually an age–sex card index with call-and-recall flagging.

While such a system is pragmatically functional, it offers little feedback to the practice concerning performance. To count the cards to get an accurate age–sex distribution at any moment in time is laborious; to assess the uptake of childhood immunisations, cervical cytology or influenza vaccines is even more so. Yet if a practice manager is to plan staffing, the doctors and nurses are to commit themselves to special screening clinics, the health visitors are to follow up all defaulters and preventive care is to become an integral part of practice life, such figures are essential. The practice must define its starting point, set objectives, formulate and implement a plan of action, and monitor progress towards the chosen goals.

There is little evidence that organised practice planning of such activity is occurring in British general practice at present, and this may be due to the widespread absence of practice statistics. Audits are time-consuming and are often performed for secondary reasons. If 'practice management' is to mean anything it must include the creation within practices of information collection systems which will be capable of supplying the necessary planning information at any time. This is an area which will be explored in Chapter 14.

In areas other than preventive care, practices do often routinely collect internal figures. Workload statistics have become more refined since they started as a simple count of patient contacts per doctor per day.[22] Many practices now collect numbers for routine surgery appointments, emergency surgery appointments, routine home visits, requested home visits and out-of-hours home visits. Such figures are of value in the planning of surgery availability, after-hours cover and for seasonal variations.

To effect change in specific areas, spasmodic data recording may be sufficient. As early as the late 1960s Practice Activity Analysis was being offered by the Birmingham Research Unit of the RCGP.[23] Participating practices were given standardised data entry sheets and were offered back their own analysis, with the average statistics of other practices for comparison. The uses of such audits have been fully described through the years;[24,25] and these can include referral rates, consulting patterns, prescribing habits, preventive uptake and investigation rates. They can be invaluable for stimulating change, but unless follow-up information gathering is undertaken such change is unlikely to be sustained.

EXTERNAL PRACTICE INFORMATION

Since the inception of the National Health Service the employing authority has supplied contracting doctors with the numbers of patients registered on their lists. This statement may appear simplistic, but it is information to which no other western primary physician has access. It is from this defined list that all the other external figures are derived, and it has fundamental implications for information gathering in general practice.

The availability of externally gathered statistics puts us in a unique position which partly explains the paucity of routine internal information gathering. If a practice can passively gain information from external sources, why should it actively collect information within the practice? The only reason is if the external information is sufficiently limited or inflexible to inhibit planning within the practice. Unfortunately this is usually the case.

Family Practitioner Committees now supply each general practitioner with information on total list sizes, the numbers of patients aged over 65 and 75, and the items-of-service claims made. This latter includes the immunisations, cervical smears, night visits, maternity fees and contraceptive fees claimed. It should be noted that the denominator population for each of these claims, except night visits, is not given, and the figures relate only to claims made and accepted. The rules governing claims for cervical cytology are so complex that, in my own practice, fewer than one in four cervical smears taken can be claimed. The FPC figures therefore give a limited picture, which is of limited value to the practice. Trends, however, may be discernible from these figures, and in the early days of quality assessments practitioners may find them useful for goal setting.

The Prescription Pricing Authority has traditionally supplied each doctor with the results of a one-month audit of the prescribing costs in a practice. The number of items prescribed, the net ingredient cost per item, the average cost per patient and the comparison of these costs to regional and national averages are given. This information is considerably more complete than the FPC returns but it is still flawed. Firstly, vocational trainees and assistants use the prescription pads of partners in the practice. Also repeat prescriptions, when written by reception staff, are often written on incorrect pads and signed by partners other than the doctor whose name appears on the prescription. The figures relate therefore to the use of that person's pad rather than his or her own specific prescribing.

Further there are questions of interpretation. Is quality greater if a small number of expensive prescriptions is issued rather than a larger number of cheaper ones? Is there any evidence to show whether cheaper prescribing is always a good concept — is there a level beneath which patient care suffers?

More detailed information is now becoming available on request from the Prescription Pricing Authority on Form PD8. The supplied information gives a breakdown by item prescribed, and can be used to look in detail at individual prescribing habits. Such information has been shown to influence prescribing habits over the short term when presented in an intelligible fashion.[26]

COMMUNITY INFORMATION

Outside primary care the quantity and quality of information improves. Hospitals and local government have been mindful of their requirements for high-quality information for decision-making for many years. Each doctor in general practice has access to information, both directly and indirectly, which can help him to plan the services he offers and to react to individual clinical situations.

Local hospitals publish outpatient waiting times, and these are usually distributed to local practices. Such figures as bed provision per thousand of population, bed occupancy, theatre throughput, admission waiting lists and community follow-up provision are available on request for each District Health Authority (DHA).

Both the DHA and local government have access to, and can supply, a breakdown for each electoral ward into age and sex, social class and deprivation indices as established in the National Census. This information is invaluable for a practice bidding, for example, for extra health visiting attachment, or planning a patient transport system. It is my experience, however, that very few practices use such information for planning purposes.

CONCLUSIONS

When faced with the increasing complexity of management tasks, many practices have set up registers which can effectively and cheaply accomplish limited objectives. While giving greater possibilities for the collation of practice statistics than the medical record envelope, manual registers are still limited in the information that they can quickly provide a practice. External sources of information may be able to supply information both about the practice and its environment, but are limited in scope and flexibility. Practice computers have been used to supply some of these functions and analyses, but these have implications in terms of cost and work efficiency.

If a practice is to develop effectively it requires detailed information on its present state and its future targets. In this review of the history of information for practice management the conclusion is drawn that such information as is required is not readily available at present.

REFERENCES

1. Jones, R.V.H., Bolden, K.J., Gray, D.J.P. and Hall, M.S. (1985) *Running a Practice*, 3rd edition. Croom Helm, London
2. Pritchard, J.M.M., Low, K. and Whalen, M. (1983) *Management in general practice*. Oxford University Press, Oxford
3. Avery Jones, Sir F. (1974) Trends in medical records. Harben Lecture
4. Martin, P., Moulds, A.J. and Kerrigan, P.J.C. (1985) *Towards better practice*. Churchill Livingstone, London
5. Pinsent, R.J.F.H. (1968) The evolving age–sex register. *Journal of the Royal College of General Practitioners*, 16, 127–34
6. Burdon, J.F. (1961) Display by spectrum. *Journal of the Royal College of General Practitioners*, 4, 106
7. Eimerl, T.S. (1960) Organized curiosity, (subtitled: A practical approach to the problem of keeping records for research purposes in general practice). *Journal of the Royal College of General Practitioners*, 3, 246–52
8. Watford, P.A. (1963) The practice index. *Journal of the Royal College of General Practitioners*, 6, 225–32
9. Morgan, R.H. (1965) The use of an age–sex register as a practice index. *Journal of the Royal College of General Practitioners*, 9, 64
10. Cooper, R.F. (1985) Do most practices have an age–sex register? Results of the West Midlands age–sex register study. *British Medical Journal*, 291, 1391–3
11. Fraser, R.C. and Clayton, D.G. (1981) The accuracy of age–sex registers, practice medical records and Family Practitioner Committee registers. *Journal of the Royal College of General Practitioners*, 31, 410–19
12. Sheldon, M.G., Rector, A.L. and Barnes, P.A. (1984) The accuracy of age–sex registers in general practice. *Journal of the Royal College of General Practitioners*, 34, 269–71
13. Royal College of General Practitioners (1963) Classification of disease. *Journal of the Royal College of General Practitioners*, 6, 219–24

14. Royal College of General Practitioners (1976) *International Classification of health problems in primary care*. Occasional Paper 1. Royal College of General Practitioners, London

15. Royal College of General Practitioners (1984) *The Classification and analysis of general practice data*. Occasional Paper 26. Royal College of General Practitioners, London

16. Crombie, D.L. (1977) Information for and from general practice. *Proceedings of the Royal Society of Medicine*, 70, 407–10

17. Walker, K. (1971) Repeat prescription recording in general practice. *Journal of the Royal College of General Practitioners*, 21, 748–51

18. Stevenson, J.S.K. (1967) Appointment systems in general practice, how patients use them. *British Medical Journal*, 2, 827–9

19. Project evaluation group (1985) *Evaluation of the 'Micros for GPs' Scheme*. HMSO, London

20. Akerman, F. (1984) Surgery computer: a quiet revolution for general practice. *British Medical Journal*, 288, 1049–53

21. Fry, J., Brooks, D. and McCall, I. (1984) *NHS Data Book*. MTP Press, Lancaster

22. Fry, J. and Dillane, J.B. (1986) Workload in a general practice 1950–85. *Journal of the Royal College of General Practitioners*, 36, 403–4

23. Royal College of General Practitioners (1973) Birmingham Research Unit and Department of Engineering Production, University of Birmingham. *Journal of the Royal College of General Practitioners*, 23, 400–3 and 404–12

24. Mourin, K. (1976) Auditing and evaluation in general practice. *Journal of the Royal College of General Practitioners*, 26, 726–33

25. Sheldon, M.G. (1981) *Medical Audit in General Practice*. Occasional Paper 20. Royal College of General Practitioners, London

26. Harris, C.M., Jarman, B., Woodman, E., White, P. and Fry, J.S. (1984) *Prescribing — a suitable case for treatment*. Occasional Paper 24. Royal College of General Practitioners, London

3

The Literature of General Practice

Simon Barley

According to Loudon,[1] the term 'general practitioner' was not seen in print until 1809. Even though for well over 100 years after that most doctors were general practitioners for at least part of their time, postgraduate training for general practice did not begin in the UK until 1946. The scientific literature of a subject grows with it; only when a branch of science has sufficient distinctiveness will there be a separate literature to describe it. In this scientific sense the specific literature of general practice could therefore start only after 1946. Before then there were few books, and no special journals whatever, for general practitioners. Ten years later a trickle had started that would grow to such a massive flood that today's chief need is for indexing and retrieval systems to allow efficient use of the literature.

BOOKS UP TO 1946

Textbooks used by doctors in training go back to Hippocrates and beyond, and presumably were the same as those used — if any — by practising doctors. Lest it be thought that these works would be few in number, it is worth noting that by the fourth century AD a vast encyclopaedia of all medical knowledge had been amassed by Oribasius, entitled *Medical collections*. C. H. Talbot, in his history of *Medicine in mediaeval England*,[2] says that this encyclopaedia, being deemed 'too unwieldy for the average practitioner', was 'summarised into nine books, reserving only those sections which would be useful to a physician living at some distance from great towns'.

The average practitioner of the Middle Ages had little need for books, but with the Renaissance and the birth of modern scientific method came the scientific journal. The first in England was the Royal Society's *Philosophical Transactions* (1665), which included medical papers, and the first purely medical journal, the Edinburgh *Medical Essays and Observations*, appeared in 1731.[3]

Loudon lists some of the many medical periodicals which sprang up between 1757 and 1866, all but eight of which have vanished, most after only a few years of publication. The *Lancet*, the *British Medical Journal* and the *Practitioner* are the survivors which are most widely read by modern general practitioners, but the *Lancet* is the only medical journal which is neither 'free' nor given away as part of the subscription to a society. It is here, in documenting the mid-nineteenth-century increase in medical literature, that it becomes apparent that there is no scholarly study of the subject. Journals wax, wane, flourish or survive, and books are published in their thousands, but I have been unable to find any articles which assess the value to the practising doctor of this monumental effort. The only evidence is inferential: publishers publish and subscribers subscribe in ever-increasing numbers, but little more can be done than to describe what was produced and to try to guess at its usefulness.

The *Medical Annual*, which started publication in 1884, attempted to keep doctors up to date in every respect, and hence a feature from the very first issue was a list of 'the most important works to the general practitioner of medicine'. There is no way of telling what the criteria for selection were, but the list ran to 12 pages in 1884–5, and was always larger thereafter.

Although so many books were published, and although until quite recently there were comparatively few specialists, it is impossible to tell how many were intended by publishers or authors for general practitioners. At least some of the works of James Mackenzie were so intended, for although in the preface to *Principles of diagnosis and treatment in heart affections* (1916)[4] he says that 'the contents . . . were prepared as lectures to be given to the postgraduate students and workers at the Cardiac Department of the London Hospital. He goes on to state that 'one of the objects I have . . . is to present the essential matters connected with heart failure in such a manner that the general practitioner can . . . apply them in his practice'. Books other than the purely clinical were also produced with the idea of helping young doctors to settle more readily and quickly into a form of medicine for which they had been little trained; five such books were *The young practitioner* (de Styrap, 1890), *An index to general practice* (A. C. Stark, 1923), *A manual of general medical practice* (W. S. Sykes, 1927), *A guide to general practice* (A. H. Douthwaite, 1932) and *Hints to the young practitioner* (G. F. Smith, 1932). This kind of guide reappeared after 1945 as Pinsent's *An approach to general practice* (1953) and Thwaite's *Into general practice* (1954); its closest relatives of the present day are the introductions to general practice written usually by academics for students (see Hammond, pp. 325–6).[5]

THE PLACE OF READING IN POSTGRADUATE EDUCATION SINCE 1950

Although the increase in the literature of general practice runs in parallel with its development as a separate branch of medicine, and the necessary defining of an education for it, it is striking how often it is assumed that reading is important in education, and yet how seldom there is any critical discussion of how and what to read.

Until the end of the 1939–45 war the general practitioner's lifetime education consisted of four elements: undergraduate teaching, refresher courses, membership of medical societies and a reading of such books and journals as were selected for study.

After the war things began to change. In 1950 a BMA Committee, chaired by Sir Henry Cohen and consisting of 35 people (only ten of whom were general practitioners), set out the first documented plan for postgraduate training in general practice.[6] A short chapter of the report was devoted in general terms to the kind of reading that general practitioners would be advised to do if their knowledge was to develop and keep up to date.

In 1952 the College of General Practitioners was founded. This step was undoubtedly the main one in establishing general practice as an independent branch of medicine, and education (with its closest relative, research) has always been one of the College's prime concerns. The impetus given by the College to postgraduate medical education (PGME) has been direct, through its reports, working parties and committees, and indirect, through the stimulation it has afforded to its members and to many other scientists inside and outside medicine. As PGME has developed one can trace the changing emphasis given to reading and going on courses, with the former almost always assumed but all too seldom given detailed consideration. Indeed some reports, even those which aim to review the whole subject of PGME, do not even mention reading. Similarly, an early attempt to establish criteria for membership did not include reading amongst desirables such as postgraduate training in hospital or in practice, going on courses and preparing case reports.[7]

An attempt to find out what general practitioners were reading appeared in 1958.[8] From a questionnaire about postgraduate study it was shown that the reading of periodicals and annuals was the most popular method, being mentioned by 99 per cent of respondents, with attendance at meetings (85 per cent), domiciliary consultations (84 per cent), reading textbooks and monographs (78 per cent) and research (26 per cent) following. The three most frequently read journals were the *British Medical Journal* (97 per cent), the *Practitioner* (72 per cent) and the *Lancet* (30 per cent).

More detail about the reading of one (albeit atypical) general practitioner was given by Fry,[9] who said that he read to keep up to date, to refresh and to revise. He read seven journals regularly. He usually borrowed a book from a library before buying it, but found that for his research and writing his own collection of books was more useful. He stated that books written for general practitioners usually sold 500–1500 per edition, a figure unchanged in 1987 (J. Fry, personal communication). He recommended that every practice should spend at least £10 for books and £10 for journals each year (the 18 books reviewed in the same issue of the College *Journal* as his article cost an average of £1.42 each, i.e. about seven books per practice per year).

Several surveys of PGME have been published in the past 20 years, and four have included questions about what GPs read.[10-13] The surveys were of different populations of doctors and did not use the same questions, so that comparisons and conclusions are hard to draw. It may be tentatively suggested on the basis of these reports that most GPs would have liked more time for reading, that most bought at least one book a year and that nearly all read one journal regularly. The most consistently popular journals have been the *British Medical Journal*, *Update*, the *Practitioner* and *Prescriber's Journal*.

Two recent studies have looked into the reading habits of general practitioners.

The first[14] describes some of the requirements of users of medical literature and how far these requirements were being met. For GPs the main reasons given for seeking information were for keeping up to date and helping with clinical problems; only 4 per cent needed it for research and 16 per cent for help with teaching (the ranking of reasons for hospital doctors was different, teaching and research figuring higher). Only 43 per cent felt they were nearly always successful in keeping up to date by meeting their information needs.

Book-buying and journal subscriptions were noted: 28 per cent of the doctors had bought no books at all in the previous year and another 36 per cent had bought only one or two, with a mere 3 per cent buying the ten or more recommended by Fry. Sixty-two per cent subscribed to one or two journals (1 per cent to five journals or more), but, presumably because so many are sent free, the number read was considerably greater. Less than one-third of the general practitioners used a medical library at least once a month, the main reason for this low figure being distance from the library. Nevertheless, time, rather than geographical situation, was felt to be the main barrier to information use.

Reviewing the above preliminary research and other data, the Medical Information Review Panel[15] recommended setting up personal links between medical librarians and general practitioners, the establishment of medically qualified Information Officers to guide general practitioners in the use of local services and wider circulation of the RCGP's *New Reading*.

BOOKS FOR GENERAL PRACTITIONERS

There is no point in merely listing the titles of the books published since 1950 and the Cohen report's adumbration of special training for general practice. An excellent survey of the literature since 1963 was made in 1984[5] by Margaret Hammond, who was appointed RCGP librarian in 1963 and who has done so much to help develop literature services for general practitioners. Altogether 210 titles are listed, most with a short description of their contents.

An attempt at a more comprehensive listing has appeared annually in the Family Medicine Literature Index (FAMLI). The lists consist of family medicine books published cumulatively in the previous three to six years, selected, according to the editors, 'on the basis of having been written by a family physician or for family physicians as the primary audience'. The listing is said to be 'comprehensive, rather than recommended', but no indication is given of the sources used. The numbers of books are given in Table 3.1, but it is not possible to say whether the increase is real or apparent. It is likely to be in part real, because in the UK the number of books for general practitioners has increased since vocational training became mandatory in 1982.

Table 3.1: New books on family medicine, 1979–85

FAMLI Year	Volume	Years included	Number of books
1981	2	1979–81	151
1982	3	1979–82	204
1983	4	1979–83	298
1984	5	1980–84	388
1985	6	1980–85	436

Two major publishers, Oxford and Churchill-Livingstone, have in the past ten years started special series on general practice, and others such as MTP Press, Tavistock publications and Croom Helm have all contributed useful titles for general practitioners. The RCGP itself has become an important publishing house, both of original books and of reports and monographs. The *Occasional Papers* series was started in 1976 and reached number 34 ten years later.

The feeling that an Oribasian universal encyclopaedia was needed became reality near the beginning of the postwar period,[16] but it has not stayed in print, nor has it been imitated since; the subject is now so large, and advancing so fast, that keeping an encyclopaedia up to date has no doubt been deemed impossible.

INDEXES, ABSTRACTING SERVICES AND BIBLIOGRAPHIES

General practitioners have always had to face the problem of information overload. In this difficulty they are no different from workers in the sciences, who have since the seventeenth century 'always felt themselves to be awash in a sea of scientific literature'. In all sciences methods designed to make the literature manageable have been developed.

Indexes

Index Medicus, a publication in monthly parts of the National Library of Medicine (Washington, USA) since 1960, is the successor to various other indexes from that Library.[17] *Index Medicus* was never published with the general practitioner particularly in mind.

In the mid-1970s Professor I. R. McWhinney began to organise a literature index of family medicine, achieving the first issue of

FAMLI (*Family Medicine Literature Index*) by 1980. It appears quarterly and in an annual cumulation. The index is in two separate sections, the first based on a modified MEDLARS search (Medicine Literature Analysis and Retrieval System) of the *Index Medicus* data base; the modification uses the standard medical subject headings, but also searches under the terms of a separately developed thesaurus of keywords commonly used in family medicine. The second section is based on a similar search of journals not indexed by *Index Medicus*. In 1986 the first part of *FAMLI* contained references culled from 2500 journals relevant to family medicine, and used 32 journals for its second part; the list of journals used for part two is constantly revised.

Abstracting services

By the early 1950s, when the College of General Practitioners was founded, the need was becoming apparent for what was at first called by Lord a Journals Monitoring Service.[18] Lord listed 13 journals which members of the College's Research Committee were already reading, and a further 13 which might be monitored. Another ten titles of free drug house publications were said 'often [to] contain worthwhile information'. Lord asked for volunteer readers to produce abstracts. One set of results was published in *Between Ourselves*, No 11, April 1959; they were unedited, and to the eye of nearly 30 years later they seem untidy, overlong and repetitive, and perhaps they did not serve the purpose, as a further selection never appeared.

Lord's early effort bore fruit in 1961, when Dr Ian Stokoe of Edinburgh began to produce *Current Medical Abstracts for Practitioners*, a quarterly publication sent free to all College members and associates. Its aim (1962 editorial) was to 'provide the practitioner with the highlights of articles that are of particular interest to him in his own sphere of work, a form of continuing postgraduate education. The abstracters were all general practitioner volunteers, and publication continued on the same basis until 1971, in which year the editor confessed to wondering 'whether it is desirable to continue with this journal when there appears to be an increasing spate of magazines, medical newspapers etc. sent free . . .'.

In 1984[19] a short report was published of a 'journal review service' organised by the Department of Postgraduate Affairs at the University of Auckland, NZ. Twenty-five general practitioner reviewers do the abstracting from 35 'relevant journals' and the results are edited, indexed and printed in a booklet sent free to every New Zealand general practitioner. A simple evaluation showed a very high level of satisfaction and perceived usefulness.

Bibliographies

The RCGP Library has produced three collections of research projects, covering the periods 1950–67, 1966–71 and 1968–73. The criteria for inclusion were slightly different in each case, and together the three volumes include many hundreds of titles.

Starting in November 1967 the *Journal of the Royal College of General Practitioners* began to publish a regular list entitled 'checklist of general-practitioner publications'. In each issue of the *Journal* 10–20 publications were given, with a one-sentence description of the contents. It is interesting to note that in November 1968 the librarian was asking readers for references to work by general practitioners on gallstones, ulcerative colitis, diverticulitis and cerebrovascular disease, as none could be found.

The next College library development to grow out of this checklist — *New Reading for General Practitioners* — was a quarterly list (cumulated annually) of articles, reports and books about general practice.

The minutes of the first meeting of the RCGP Library Committee (October, 1958) record the intention that *eventually* (their italics) the Library should contain everything written about general practice and everything written on medical subjects by general practitioners. In 1960 the first librarian was appointed, and by 1961 she reported that 506 requests for bibliographies were being met each month. This service to individual College members has continued ever since.

Conclusion

No satisfactory single source of abstracts, bibliographies or indexing can yet be recommended for general practitioners. *FAMLI* is very comprehensive, but misses the unusual or out-of-the-way reports that do not feature in journals or books, and *New Reading* (or, to give it its grand new title, 'RCGP Information Resources Centre list of publications on general practice') is 'not comprehensive'.

LEARNED JOURNALS OF GENERAL PRACTICE

As the association journal of a professional body founded by general practitioners and always including most of the profession's GPs as members, the *British Medical Journal* has always been an important medium in which GPs could read and write their views. The correspondence columns in particular are the best barometer of general practitioner opinion and must always be one of the historian's prime sources for the profession's views on the issues of the day. Nevertheless, just as other specialties have started their own journals, so general practice needed to do the same, and in 1958 the College of General Practitioners issued volume one of the world's first journal of general practice. The aim of this journal has always been to concentrate on publishing original research papers,[20,21] an achievement which had led it to become the most cited general practice journal after the US *Journal of Family Practice* (1974-   ).[22]

The history of the RCGP's journal has been written.[23] It is sufficient to say here that it obviously filled an enormous need in its early days. Not only was it the embodiment of one of the original projects contained in the College's Memorandum of Association (to publish original research) but it also served to channel what Murray-Scott called 'all this bottled-up curiosity released by the [College's] research committee'. The research committee had also been responsible for the forerunners of the *Journal*, the two informal publications called *Between Ourselves* (1956–67) and *Research Newsletter* (1953–60). Another information publication of the research committee, *Progress Reports*, was absorbed into *Between Ourselves* in October 1956. The first five issues of the *Research Newsletter* were published in the *Practitioner*, itself an important journal for general practitioners, and a strong supporter of the College.

No other research journal of general practice was started in the UK until the WONCA-sponsored quarterly *Family Practice* appeared in 1984. Edited by Professor John Howie of Edinburgh, its editorial board is an impressive list of internationally respected teachers of general practice, and has concentrated on longer papers.

Journals of family medicine and general practice have become established gradually in many other countries, but the present chapter must necessarily concentrate on the United Kingdom.

NEWSPAPERS AND MAGAZINES FOR GENERAL PRACTITIONERS AND REVIEW JOURNALS

In his classic essay on the medical journal and its future, Fox[24] identified two contrasting types — the *medical recorder* (noting new observations, experiments and techniques and being the principal means of communication between investigators) and the *medical newspaper*, which informs, interprets, criticises, stimulates and by telling doctors what other doctors are doing helps to integrate the profession. Although there has obviously been much of the medical newspaper in the *Lancet* and *BMJ* ever since they started, medical newspapers were pioneered from about 1950 in the USA with the first — *Pulse* — appearing in the UK in 1959; the other two weeklies surviving in 1987 are *General Practitioner* (1963) and *Doctor* (1971).

The only detailed consideration of these and the many other medical newspapers which have come and gone since 1959 is by Cowhig,[25] himself the editor of *General Practitioner*. He pointed out that what he called a gigantic phenomenon (in 1981 £21 million was spent in buying advertising space) was remarkably little recorded, an omission that has still to be rectified in 1987. Cowhig's discussion remains the sole contribution in the medical literature describing in any detail the characteristics of the main publications in the 'GP market'. They are widely circulated and read; they compete for readership and advertising, on which they rely for their income, and they are distributed free. Although total advertising income has diminished since its peak in 1981, when *Pulse* and *General Practitioner* ran to about 100 pages each week, the distribution of readership is still much the same (allowing for some losses, e.g. of *World Medicine*). The content, however, has changed. In 1965, soon after it was launched, a typical issue of *General Practitioner* (known simply as *GP* then) carried one case report, one article about a new diuretic called Lasix, another about osteopathy and eleven non-clinical items on motoring, travel, politics and so on. *Pulse* had virtually no clinical material whatever, but a great deal of medico-political news and comment. The first issue of *Doctor* (14 January 1971) carried the managing director's statement recommending his paper's range of services for readers including financial and leisure advice, news of advances in medicine and medical politics; one only of the 16 pages in that first issue was clinical. The weeklies now give doctors professional, well-designed and well-produced papers which, according to Cowhig, almost all doctors read sometimes.

The magazines are virtually synonymous with the review journals. *World Medicine* was an important exception. It was launched in 1965 with an impressive masthead. Edited at first by Dr Donald Gould, its heyday was the ten years when it was the fortnightly child of Dr Michael O'Donnell, a general practitioner turned campaigning journalist of genius, who succeeded in using his magazine to fight for reform of the General Medical Council. When the magazine was sold, and O'Donnell resigned, it limped on for a year or two and disappeared.

Whereas O'Donnell, if challenged, would probably have said that he had no policy except to publish interesting articles about medical matters that doctors wanted to read, the next influential journal to be started — *Update* — always had a self-consciously higher policy — postgraduate education for general practitioners. Its first editor was another doctor-journalist, Abraham Marcus, who shrewdly saw that the movement to build postgraduate centres which stemmed from Sir George Pickering's 1961 conference at Christ Church College, Oxford, could support a journal 'founded to serve this movement in every way possible' (Editorial to volume 1, number 1, October 1968). Marcus chose John Fry as his editorial adviser, with a widely cast net drawing in general practitioners of all kinds, for his editorial board. Like *World Medicine*, *Update* was a fortnightly magazine of high-quality printing, writing and production standards (especially illustrations). It contained little original material, but concentrated on printing lectures given by specialists and, in later years, inventively titled series of articles reflecting themes encountered by general practitioners in everyday practice — prescribing, diagnosis, management, minor surgery, the difficult or rare cases and so on. *Update* has remained a professional and widely read publication, successful enough for several other journals to be launched on its back — *Trainee* (1981–), *Medical Teacher* (1979–) and others for hospital doctors and dentists. Update publications also published the *Journal of the Royal College of General Practitioners* from 1977 to 1983.

There have been several other fortnightly or monthly free magazines but although some are distinctive (e.g. *MIMS Magazine*, devoted entirely to therapeutics) there is insufficient space in which to discuss them here, and in any case they are largely unobtainable for study as libraries very rarely file them. One publication, *Prescriber's Journal*, must be considered because of its longevity (1961), because it is so widely read and because it has therefore been an important source of information for general practitioners. *Prescriber's Journal*, preceded by *Prescriber's Notes* from 1952 to 1961, is published by the Department of Health and Social Security (DHSS) six times a year, and is devoted entirely to therapeutics. Being small in format and thickness, and lacking advertisements, it is completely different from all the unsolicited offerings supported by the pharmaceutical industry. Its articles are short, authoritative and usually well written (but unillustrated), so that careful and continual reading should in theory keep doctors up to date. The DHSS plainly thinks it has the product about right, since the style and format have altered very little over the years; it has also had the same editor, J. L. Hunt, from the beginning.

The DHSS also supports another fortnightly publication on therapeutics, the *Drug and Therapeutics Bulletin* (*DTB*) published by the Consumers' Association. *DTB* began in 1963 and was available only by subscription until 1980, when the DHSS instituted its free distribution to every general practitioner working in the National Health Service. Its editor, A. Herhexheimer, has also been in charge since its inception, but his perspective, that of an academic clinical pharmacologist, has been different both from DHSS and from drug-industry supported publications, and the *DTB* is nearer in philosophy and style to the publications of its parent body. Its tone is sceptical and critical, and it is reluctant to accept claims for drugs that are supported by anything but the most scientifically irreproachable evidence.

Health Trends, also published by the DHSS, must be mentioned, but as it is sent to all NHS doctors it is not designed especially for general practitioners.

CONCLUSIONS: HOW MUCH DO GENERAL PRACTITIONERS READ?

This historical survey of information sources for general practitioners has inevitably been discursive and descriptive only: there are remarkably few salient facts in these matters. The predominant impression gained by someone studying the subject is the lack of research. Books and journals are published and distributed in huge quantities, but nobody knows how much they are read and, more important, how much they are used in day-to-day practice. This field is undoubtedly not an easy one in which to do research, and some speculation is therefore in order.

Fox, quoting J. D. Bernal, the physicist who tried throughout his life to reform and rationalise scientific communication, says that 'practical scientists do not read much anyway', and A. Gillie, the only woman president of the RCGP (1964–7) said[26] 'the full educational scope and its demands that face us today has little reality for many among the mature and *often very weary doctors* in practice' (italics added). If the sheer exhausting pressure of work — and what Dr John Stevens of Aldeburgh called 'being battered by the commonplace' — is one reason why doctors do not read, are there others? Some are suggested in a penetrating chapter by Bloom,[27] who discusses the relationship between what doctors experience as students and what they actually do having graduated. One study quoted by Bloom suggests that students, although intelligent and curious about their future career, were nevertheless basically practical in their orientation towards it; they were 'training for uncertainty',[28] and Thomson has suggested[29] that general practitioners, more than other doctors, learn in their work to tolerate uncertainty. The certainty of books is the very antithesis of the uncertainty of daily practice, and I suggest that general practitioners, although they must obviously create and sustain a basis of factual knowledge for their work, must also learn to balance these facts with daily experiences that are at variance with them. There are several other factors that make general practitioners prone to use their wits rather than written sources: they practise rapidly and in such a way that their patient, rather than asking for 'the answer' at once, can, by repeated visits, be allowed to demonstrate the evolution of the illness spontaneously — the patient provides the answer, not necessarily the doctor or the books; they are flooded with prescriptive information, so that skipping through a review article becomes a substitute for hard study and revision; they can, if they do not know something, almost invariably refer their patient to someone who does, so that there is no premium on finding out for oneself; the field of work in which they are required to make decisions is so vast that again it is tempting to decide that one will keep a wide working knowledge at one's fingertips rather than become an expert in detail; and finally, teaching and research are minority pursuits.

It remains to be seen whether any of these constraints will be overcome by the new methods of acquiring, storing and retrieving information.

REFERENCES

1. Loudon, I. (1986) *Medical care and the general practitioner 1750–1850*. Oxford University Press, Oxford
2. Talbot, C.H. (1967) *Medicine in mediaeval England*. Oldbourne, London
3. Booth, C.C. (1982) Medical communication: the old and the new. The development of medical journals in Britain. *British Medical Journal*, 285, 105–8
4. Mackenzie, J. (1916) *Principles of diagnosis and treatment in heart affections*. Oxford Medical Publications, London
5. Hammond, M. (1984) General practice. In: Morton, L.T. and Godbolt, S. (eds), *Information sources in the medical sciences*. Butterworths, London, pp. 321–37
6. British Medical Association (1950) *General practice and the training of the general practitioner* (Cohen report). BMA, London
7. Hunt, J.H. (1964) Criteria for membership. *Journal of the College of General Practitioners*, 7, 139–43
8. College of General Practitioners (1958) Analysis of replies to a questionnaire from the Postgraduate Education Committee of Council. 4: Postgraduate study for principals. *Journal of the College of General Practitioners*, 1, 171–5
9. Fry, J. (1965) Books and the general practitioner. *Journal of the College of General Practitioners*, 10, 309–10
10. Byrne, P.S. (1969) Preparation for teaching in general practice. *Journal of the Royal College of General Practitioners*, 17, 69–79
11. Acheson, H.W.K. (1974) Continuing education in general practice in England and Wales. *Journal of the Royal College of General Practitioners*, 24, 643–7
12. Durno, D. and Gill, G.M. (1974) Survey of general practitioners' views on postgraduate education in N.E. Scotland. *Journal of the Royal College of General Practitioners*, 24, 648–54
13. Pickings, A.J., Mee, L.G. and Hedley, A.J. (1983) The general practitioner and continuing education. *Journal of the Royal College of General Practitioners*, 33, 486–90
14. Ford, G., Maguire, V. and Palmer, P. (1980) The use of medical literature: a preliminary survey. (British Library research and development report No. 5515). British Library, London
15. Cockerill, P.E. (1981) Information and the practice of medicine. British Library research and development report No. 5605. British Library, London
16. Abercrombie, G.F. and McConaghey, R.M.S. (eds) (1963) *Encyclopaedia of general practice*. Butterworths, London
17. Sutherland, F.M. (1974) Indexes, abstracts, bibliographies and reviews. In Morton, L.T. (ed.), *Use of medical literature*. Butterworths, London, vol. 4, pp. 34–57
18. Lord, W.J.H. (1957) A journals monitoring service. *Between Ourselves*, (no date, probably 1957): *4* (late extra), 4–10

19. Benseman, J. and Barham, P.M. (1984) Coping with information overload: the development and evaluation of a journal review service. *Medical Education*, *18*, 446–7

20. Editorial (1969) Why a College Journal? *Journal of the Royal College of General Practitioners*, *17*, 1–2

21. Editorial (1980) What kind of Journal? *Journal of the Royal College of General Practitioners*, *30*, 707–9

22. Geyman, J.P. (1983) Citation analysis of *The Journal of Family Practice*. *Journal of Family Practice*, *16*, 812–19

23. Pereira Gray, D.J. (1983) The College Journal. In: Fry J., Lord Hunt of Fawley and Pinsent, R.J.F.H. (eds), *A history of the Royal College of General Practitioners: the first 25 years*. MTP, Lancaster, 160–7

24. Fox, T.F. (1965) *Crisis in Communication*. Athlone Press, London

25. Cowhig, J. (1982) The medical newspaper. *British Medical Journal*, *285*, 109–11

26. Gillie, A. (1964) Reflections on the Gillie report. *Journal of the Royal College of General Practitioners*, *7*, 1–8

27. Bloom, S.W. (1980) The process of becoming a physician and the context of medical education. In: Noack, H. (ed.), *Medical education and primary health care*. Croom Helm, London, pp. 144–60

28. Fox, R. (1957) Training for uncertainty. In: Merton, R.K., Leader, G.C. and Kendall, P.L. (eds), *The student physician*. University Press, Cambridge, Mass., 207–41

29. Thomson, G.H. (1978) Tolerating uncertainty in family medicine. *Journal of the Royal College of General Practitioners*, *28*, 343–6

4

Information for Patients

Susan Clayton

Do general practitioners provide written information to their patients? What type of information is available to GPs to distribute? How adequate is this material and how well is it distributed?

GPs are frequently encouraged to distribute written information to their patients but it is necessary to ask whether GPs are heeding that advice, and whether the quality of material available for distribution is satisfactory. To help answer these questions this chapter outlines the range of written information typically available to patients in the surgeries of British general practitioners, and then evaluates its quality and systems of distribution. This is then followed by a discussion of some factors inhibiting the use of written material as a means of offering information to patients.

PERSONAL AND PRE-PREPARED MATERIAL

Patients require many different types of information, including details of how to manage their disorder and promote their own health. Traditionally most of this information has been given to patients verbally. Increasingly, however, the limitations to this method of communication have been recognised. In particular it is considered inappropriate to expect patients to recall accurately complex information which has only been given to them verbally. In some circumstances it is also considered poor use of a doctor's time to explain background information which might more usefully be written down and given to the patient for reference if and when appropriate.[1-3]

Two different types of written information can be identified. One is information prepared specifically for an individual patient (for example a letter explaining the diagnosis of the patient's condition) and the other pre-prepared material designed for certain categories of patient (for example a leaflet encouraging smokers to stop smoking).

There is little evidence of general practitioners writing down information or instructions for individual patients. GPs tend to rely on the spoken word for giving specific information to individual patients, although a few give patients some jottings on a piece of paper, and there is some use of quasi-personal letters to ask patients to attend the surgery or to let them know test results. Even though GPs, on referring patients to hospital consultants, write a letter about the patient's situation it is unusual for patients to be shown this.

In contrast to the lack of material written specially for a single patient, general practitioners make considerable use of pre-prepared material. They often find it useful to give such literature to patients and relatives for subsequent reading and reference. The rest of this chapter focuses upon this type of written literature, although with the coming of word processors the distinction between pre-prepared information and that written for a specific patient will soften.

Attention will now be paid to: (1) material pre-prepared for patients on the treatment and care of specific medical conditions; (2) prescribed drugs; (3) health promotion; (4) operation of GP practices; (5) the role of other health and welfare agencies, and (6) patients' rights.

1. Treatment and care of specific medical conditions

Specific information about the medical condition of a patient is mostly transmitted in the consultation via the spoken word, plus non-verbal communication such as eye contact and body language. However, increasingly GPs are reinforcing their message by giving patients written information on their condition and its management, and its implications for their own and their family's future well-being.

The material that GPs offer patients comes from a variety of sources, especially commercial pharmaceutical companies and voluntary organisations. A small number of practices prepare their own leaflets, and the Health Education Council, although primarily focusing on health promotion, also produces a little material on the treatment of medical conditions. A few practices run their own patient lending libraries.

The quality of material available for GPs to distribute to patients varies enormously. Much material is well produced and sensitive to the likely needs of readers. Some, however, reads as though it has been thrown together with little concern for the needs of the reader or the variety of different experiences of those who may be given the leaflet. It has also to be recognised that the production of patient leaflets sometimes forms part of a commercial company's advertising strategy, and that the information given may present only a limited perspective.

A problem with many of these leaflets is that they are written in language which is too complex. On the other hand some leaflets can be criticised for being so short and simple that they offer too little information.

Despite these criticisms there is much good material available for GPs to give to patients. Problems, however, often occur with the distribution of such material. There is no easy method by which GPs can learn of and evaluate the wealth of potentially valuable information for patients. It is time-consuming and costly for GPs to select, order and manage the mass of excellent leaflets they could appropriately distribute to patients. Instead it appears that most GPs operate in a rather *ad hoc* manner. For example, if leaflets are sent to the surgery these may be displayed in the waiting room until stocks run down, but few attempts are made specifically to order supplies of suitable literature for each major client group.

2. Information about prescribed drugs

When patients are prescribed a drug by their GP they get some written instructions on the package and sometimes a written 'patient package insert'. These inserts tend either to be absent or to contain a mass of complex technical information presented in small print. As a consequence many patients either receive no information, or material which is difficult to understand and to pull out points of direct relevance. Some good leaflets are available for GPs or pharmacists to hand to patients, but few have filtered through to the GP surgery.

3. Health promotion

A great deal of well-presented information is published which aims at encouraging people to lead healthier lifestyles. This is supplemented by contributions from commercial and voluntary organisations. Occasionally health education material is printed in the languages of relevant ethnic minorities, and a few practices run video or tape–slide programmes in their waiting room to supplement written health promotion messages.

Some of the best written material available for patients comes from the Health Education Authority. Most of their leaflets and posters are well written and cleverly illustrated. They also tend to exhibit sensitivity to important issues such as race and gender; for example including portrayals of women in non-standard roles and illustrations of black people. The quality of material from other sources varies enormously, some being excellent, some very poorly written and reproduced.

Major problems arise with the funding of health promotional leaflets. Voluntary organisations producing leaflets have only limited budgets, and even the Health Education Council's publications have sometimes to be rationed. As with the supply of leaflets on the management of medical conditions, there are also serious problems with managing the supply of leaflets in doctors' surgeries and of ensuring that suitable leaflets reach target audiences.

4. The existence of GP surgeries and details of their operation

Slowly the needs of patients to know basic information about GP practices are being recognised formally. There is now greater awareness of the benefit of helping patients identify which GPs accept patients from a particular geographical locality, and helping patients to learn how each of these practices operates (for example when they are open, how a doctor should be called out in an emergency, whether there is a practice nurse or well-woman clinic).

Increasingly GPs are preparing their own 'patient information' leaflet containing information about the operation of their practice. A small number also produce regular newsletters or an annual report which gives information about the practice and its policies, and healthy living. The standard of 'patient information' leaflets varies enormously. Some are excellent, especially where patients or professional writers are involved in their production, but rather too many forget to include important information for patients, such as how to reach the surgery and where the nearest bus stops are located. Furthermore there often appears little enthusiasm for making sure that these leaflets and their updates are made available to all patients.

In the past the giving of information about practices to patients was bedevilled by doctors' fears that they would be charged with malpractice if they gave information to patients which might be construed as advertising. However, in 1986 the General Medical Council changed its guidance to doctors and encouraged the production of factual information on practice management and facilities. Family Practitioner Committees were also encouraged to improve the availability and usability of lists of local general practitioners.

Despite these changed guidelines on practice administration, the question of making available information to patients about doctors' activities remains controversial. For example, some people argue that to tell patients of the goals of a practice is to advertise. Others suggest that it is acceptable to tell patients the aims of the practice but not the extent to which these goals are being met. Supporters of making information more available to patients suggest that fears of advertising are dominating the debate to the detriment of the needs of patients. They also suggest that it is only right and proper that patients should be able to learn of the activities of their doctors, and to hold them accountable for their behaviour.

5. Information about other health and welfare services

General practitioners play a key role in referring patients to other statutory and voluntary services providing health and welfare services. Formal referrals tend to take place via telephone or letter from the GP to the agency involved. However, there are occasions when the GP recommends that a patient approaches an agency but leaves him or her to make the contact. In some of these cases the GP gives the patient a leaflet explaining the role of the recommended agency and how it can be contacted. In other cases patients learn of voluntary organisations of potential value to themselves via leaflets, posters or directories displayed in the waiting room.

The availability of such leaflets in GP practices tends to be poor. Like other written patient information sent to doctors, they may be unsolicited, and if felt to be useful displayed in the surgery, but rarely is there a systematic scheme for selecting suitable leaflets or ensuring that exhausted stocks are recorded.

Unfortunately while directories of local services, both statutory and voluntary, are often produced by local agencies, these do not appear to be readily available in GP practices, despite their potential benefit both to patients and doctor. Furthermore, while details of voluntary organisations and statutory services are available on certain computer-based data banks these tend not to be accessible direct from the surgery.

6. Patients' rights

A few surgeries display leaflets or posters about the rights of patients prepared by such organisations as the National Consumer Council or local Community Health Council. In general, however, it seems that little information of this nature is available. It is therefore often hard for patients to learn (for example) arrangements for second opinions or changing doctor, or how to make a formal complaint about their GP.

While GPs recognise the correlation between poverty and ill-health only a limited number display Department of Health and Social Security and local government leaflets on welfare benefits.

LIMITATIONS IN THE USE OF WRITTEN INFORMATION

The above outline of availability of written information by general practitioners to patients suggests that provision of such material is limited and poorly organised, despite encouragement to GPs to give patients such information. While this is disappointing, the picture does seem to be improving: much more material appears to be produced for, and displayed in, GP surgeries than even a few years ago.

The increased availability of written information in GP surgeries is to be welcomed, but there are a number of factors which appear to be inhibiting the development of comprehensive systems of written information. These are now outlined.

It would appear that many patients have low expectations of written information from their GP. It is perhaps surprising that patients did not complain more bitterly in the past about the lack of written information available to them on practice facilities. Similarly one might have expected more criticism of the lack of provision of helpful leaflets on treatment made available to them via their GP. Patients expect verbal advice from their doctor, but as yet they do not appear to expect written information advising them how to manage their condition or to prevent its recurrence.

Many doctors appear to give low priority to the provision of written information to their patients. They recognise its value but feel their limited time is more appropriately spent in other directions. Unfortunately it does take time to organise good schemes, and such work has to compete with other activities which often seem more urgent or important. Even when doctors do make time within the practice to prepare material, the leaflets and posters may be drawn up primarily with the doctor's interests in mind, rather than patients'. The material produced or displayed, and its content, may reflect what the doctor wishes his or her patients to know, not what the latter particularly desire information on. Thus, for example, a practice management leaflet may stress the importance of patients not requesting a home visit other than when absolutely essential, or not requesting surgery appointments on a Saturday. Basic information of interest to patients, such as the location of the surgery, the geographical areas from which patients will be taken on, and whether there is a patients' toilet on the premises, may be missing.

Arrangements which keep written information about a patient secret from the person involved may also be seen as assisting the doctor rather more than the patient. Certainly in many cases important channels of written communication are missed because patients do not have access to their own file, or letters to and from consultants. Of course some patients manage to read their case notes, or dare to steam open letters they have been asked to take to the hospital. However, even in these circumstances they may learn relatively little, as the information is not written with their needs in mind.

In considering why patient-oriented information is inadequate it has to be recognised that lack of information to patients tends to increase their anxiety while enhancing the power of the doctor. One of the characteristics of professions is a desire to keep a tight rein on information in order to maintain a monopoly over certain knowledge. Thus while doctors may speak of the benefits of giving patients increased information, in reality they may feel ambivalent about this activity and reluctant to give up their power.

Even where there is a genuine commitment to producing written material, problems can occur. The cost of production tends to encourage the design of only a limited number of short documents. However, one brief leaflet on a condition is unlikely to cover the interests of all interested readers — for example children and adults, new cases and people who have had the condition for many years.

Some people want basic information, others are relatively well educated about their condition and want detailed information on self-management. The case for different leaflets for different audiences is persuasive, but the logistical and financial consequences of this can be enormous.

Many leaflets given to patients miss valuable opportunities to transmit useful information because they are poorly produced. GPs and those assisting them may lack the skills and time to prepare good material. Certainly some of the poorest-quality patient information material is that produced by GP practices or small organisations who are well-meaning but have not given the necessary time to identifying what patients wish to know, nor have they the resources to prepare well-informed, easy-to-read, attractive material. It is salutary also to note that even when specialist advice is available on presenting information, for example from the Campaign for Plain English, relatively few people appear to be aware of such help, or willing to spend time and money capitalising on this expertise.

Allied to lack of motivation to produce good written material for patients is unwillingness to allocate the necessary resources to this activity. It takes money to produce leaflets and to pay staff to administer schemes. Many GPs appear reluctant to spend money in this way, partly because there are few pressures on them to make this investment and also because they are not specifically refunded for this activity.

Excellent publications of both simple and sophisticated design are often available for purchase from relevant voluntary organisations or bookshops, but there is no special funding for GPs to purchase these for free distribution to patients, and no system for ordering them for patients 'on prescription'. Similarly, while charitable organisations often wish to distribute their material free, they too are constrained in their activities by financial factors.

LIMITATIONS IN THE ORGANISATION OF WRITTEN INFORMATION

It is not only a case of insufficient interest in, and lack of money for, producing written information for patients, but also inadequate commitment to setting up systems for the management of written material. Vast amounts of written material are available to GPs for potential distribution to appropriate patients, but the sources of these are numerous and often difficult to identify. Furthermore, the quality of material available varies greatly. Ideally much time is required to identify and evaluate potential material. Most GPs do not feel they have the time available to carry out this activity.

A good system of patient information also requires constant management. After suitable free leaflets have been selected they have to be ordered, displayed and restocked. Suitable display shelves or racks have also to be identified, purchased and maintained. Ideally special attempts need to be made to reach adolescent patients, elderly patients and patients with reading difficulties with suitable material.

Unfortunately there is little impetus for GPs to correct a poor situation; perhaps because the mass of potentially useful material is large and there is so little assistance for them in this task. It is perhaps unreasonable, and wasteful of human resources, to expect every practice to take on all this by themselves. Tasks such as the identification and evaluation of leaflets might well be carried out by a central organisation or by Family Practitioner Committees.

Some assistance is available to GPs, for example an occasional article in a medical magazine which lists a selection of patient information leaflets. However, these lists tend to be limited in range and some are biased towards leaflets produced by commercial companies. Neither the Department of Health and Social Security nor individual Family Practitioner Committees appear to offer much assistance to GPs, although they sometimes send out bundles of useful literature. It is rare to see serious reviews of patient information literature in the professional press, and there is no central store from which GPs can order a wide range of free patient information leaflets.

CONCLUSIONS

The range of patient information literature available from GP surgeries appears to be growing, but still to be very limited in quantity and poorly administered. This occurs despite considerable encouragement to doctors to give written information to appropriate patients. The poor use of such material is unfortunate, as general practitioners are ideally placed to provide patients with suitable material. On average patients visit their GP four times a year,[4] and most could therefore be exposed regularly to displays of health education literature. GP surgeries also provide an excellent location for the display of welfare rights material, especially health-related leaflets about schemes to assist with the cost of fares to hospital, medicines and spectacles. The personal contact and rapport between GP and patient also provides a good opportunity for patients to be handed appropriate written advice on their medical condition, and encouragement to heed the advice given.

Currently, spoken communication takes high precedence over written information. Patients have low expectations of the latter, and GPs give its provision low priority, especially when the multiplicity of sources makes identification of appropriate literature difficult and time-consuming.

The value of using written material as a medium for communication is, however, increasingly being recognised by doctors and patients alike, and the quality and quantity of such material is improving. Many GPs want to improve their provision of written information to patients and are seeking assistance with the logistics of the exercise. They need encouragement to solve their difficulties, and probably also help from outside sources. Some patient participation groups make a good contribution in this area, and computerisation of information can help enormously. Nonetheless the task of identifying potentially useful information, and ensuring that patients receive appropriate material, is daunting. Much assistance has been given to GPs towards improving the standard of their verbal communication with patients. The time is now ripe to assist them with the presentation of written material.

ACKNOWLEDGEMENT

The author would like to thank Dr Peter Pritchard for the kind support and assistance that he gave towards the preparation of this chapter.

REFERENCES

1. Ley, P. (1983) Patients' understanding and recall in clinical communication failure. In: Pendleton, D. and Hasler, J. (eds), *Doctor-patient communication*. Academic Press, London
2. Gann, R. (1986) *The health information handbook, resources for self care*. Gower, Aldershot
3. Clayton, S. (1986) Prescribing information to patients. *British Medical Journal*, 292, 1368
4. Office of Population, Census and Surveys (1983) *General Household Survey*. HMSO, London

5

A Review of Information for People

Richard Westcott

At the beginning of this century there was little information readily available to the lay public in Britain on health or illness. Today the amount of accessible information is enormous. In this chapter the way in which health information has increased and diffused through society will be described. In contrast to information for patients dealt with in the previous chapter the scene here is society as a whole, away from the general practitioner, the surgery and the health centre.

One theme which runs through this account is that the role of the medical profession has, on the whole, been less than glorious. Although the behaviour of most doctors has exemplified Bernard Shaw's remark that 'all professions are conspiracies against the laity' a few have, often with evangelical fervour, tried to spread information against the wishes of their colleagues.

EARLY BEGINNINGS

One early work which contained much health and hygiene information was *The constitution of man*, published by George Combe, a phrenologist, in 1828. Although before 1830 sources of reference were available in libraries for those who could, or wished to, read they were distanced from most people as well as being expensive. At about this time a movement arose which lobbied Parliament with fervour to incorporate the teaching of hygiene in educational reform.

The earliest health leaflets for general distribution were produced during the three great cholera epidemics, the first in 1831.[1] These leaflets were a factor in the establishment of sanitary and other enabling legislation which brought about huge improvements in standards of living. Infectious diseases were combated, nutrition improved and disease patterns changed.[2]

The period 1830–70 was one in which there was 'strenuous campaigning for health.[1] Signs of this ferment include the foundation of the Health of Towns Association (1842), the Epidemiological Society (1850) and the Sanitary Association of Manchester and Salford (1852), whose ladies section pioneered the use of health visiting. The Ladies Physiological Reform Society dared to broach the topics of female anatomy and physiology.[3] The Anti-Tobacco Society was formed. Throughout Britain local public health services slowly became established. First Aid became a subject for lectures and examinations.

Accompanying this activity printed material concerned with hygiene and health steadily expanded. In 1835 Hodgkin produced *The means of promoting and preserving health*, the first such text of substance. In America Sylvester Graham, a Pennsylvanian temperance lecturer, inspired the Popular Health Movement, lectured widely and wrote *The home book of life and health*. The societies which were formed themselves produced pamphlets and books. Information appeared as a by-product of other activities — for example as part of the fund-raising efforts to establish the Great Ormond Street Hospital a manual was published in 1854 on how to nurse sick children, 'intended especially as a help to the Nurses at the Hospital for Sick Children but also containing directions which may be found of service to all who have charge of the Young'.[4] In this publication there are clear descriptions of the infectious diseases of childhood, with diagnostic and therapeutic points helpfully explained in simple language for the laity.

Such educational efforts, by individuals and by 'associations of citizens intent on public enlightenment', tended to be discouraged and even opposed outright by doctors. Graham's Popular Health Movement in America developed along anti-medical lines with emphasis on Good Living as contrasted to the need for orthodox medical care. The setting up of Florence Nightingale's training school for nurses provides another example which illustrates the unwillingness of the medical profession to share its knowledge, and demonstrating the opposition which the medical establishment could muster. After the Resident Medical Officer and Matron had committed St Thomas' to the new scheme, the Senior Surgeon, Mr J. F. South (President of the Royal College of Surgeons), reacted so strongly that he published a book in 1857 in which 'he argued that nurses were subordinates "in the position of housemaids" and needed only the simplest instruction, such as how to make a poultice'.[5]

Florence herself thundered back, in her *Notes on Nursing* (1859):

> It is constantly objected — 'But how can I obtain this medical knowledge? I am not a doctor. I must leave this to doctors'. Oh, mothers of families! . . . Is all this premature suffering and death necessary? Or did Nature intend mothers to be always accompanied by doctors? Or is it better to learn the piano-forte than to learn the laws which subserve the preservation of offspring? . . . Extraordinary is it that, whereas what we call the coxcombries of education — eg the elements of astronomy — are now taught to every school girl, neither mothers of families of any class, nor school mistresses of any class, nor nurses . .. are taught anything about those laws . . . of life. They call it medical or physiological knowledge, fit only for doctors.[6]

1870–1920

By 1870 the elements of health education were beginning to diffuse more widely, on a national rather than parochial basis. Popular medical dictionaries for home and family use started to appear. Lectures and examinations led to the granting of First Aid Certificates in 1877. The first manual of instruction in First Aid was published in 1878. This aspect of health care was especially keenly taken up by miners, policemen and railwaymen, with 400 classes being established within the first three years. *Aids for cases of injuries or sudden illness* was frequently rewritten, re-edited and republished over the next ten years in response to public demand.

In the public domain three out of every five volunteers for Boer War Service were found to be unfit to serve. Increasing awareness of the extent of poor health among the nation at large was the stimulus behind the Report on National Physical Deterioration.

The years leading up to the First World War saw rapid changes in society. Systematic elementary education, the establishment of the Labour Party and the development of the Workers' Educational Association all contributed to a real democratisation of Britain, represented by an extra 8,500,000 on the electoral register. There was a wave of strikes with demands for 'freedom' (be it for workers, women or Ireland), and emancipation was in the air. The new power-sharing demanded information-sharing.

The First World War accelerated these changes. Health leaflets, lectures and posters about illness prevention, slogans, Health Weeks and cigarette-type health cards, were part of everyday life.

The war had introduced millions of men to the sheath, the diaphragm was invented at the same time and Marie Stopes' pioneering *Married Love* was published in 1918. But it was to be a further 12 years before the Ministry of Health was to allow birth control instruction, and then only for mothers who were considered to need it on medical grounds. There were individual doctor educators, no doubt, but it seems as though the profession in general was more concerned with maintaining restrictions despite (or because of) the growth of the media, extensions of the franchise, educational improvements and accelerating changes in society.

Throughout this period the number of health reports from official sources also increased, and slowly became the norm. An example of this practice is the *Annual Report from the Medical Officers of Health for North Devon and Exeter*,[7] published by Devon County Council in 1907/8. In this report, alongside local birth and death rates, can be found comments on the state of schools, of factories and housing. Positive suggestions are made about practical steps which could be taken to improve people's health. Sound medical and health information was now being addressed to county councillors: it was no longer a case of just the evangelisers, zealots and enthusiasts, but managers, state employees and business people needing and wanting to know.

1920–THE PRESENT

Radio began in 1922. Television was established in 1936. Since 1920 voluntary organisations and official bodies, although continuing to publish books, pamphlets and articles, have become increasingly involved in exploiting these two media for health education. During this time health and illness have become matters of interest, even of absorbing fascination to the population at large — and information about them has become a commercial commodity. Health information, seductively packaged, sells magazines and newspapers, and attracts people to watch television.

Voluntary organisations

Voluntary organisations and self-help groups have largely stayed loyal to printed matter. They have issued leaflets and books. New associations have sprung up to meet the needs of particular groups stimulated by failure of the Health Service to do so.

A recent example is the formation of BACUP (The British Association of Cancer United Patients and their families and friends) in 1986 to provide information and support. The contribution made by these groups and organisations in presenting information on health and illness direct to the public is enormous with some, such as the British Diabetic Association, being pre-eminent.

Perhaps because in only a minority of such organisations doctors have been involved in their formation, their self-help qualities are accompanied by spontaneity, vitality, innovativeness and flexibility.[8] Although they may have subsequently co-operated closely with, and sometimes have been led by, doctors they are essentially lay organisations finding their cohesion in a shared experience or vision, characteristics which pervade their literature.

Official bodies

As in the First World War, the Second saw a great increase of government spending on health education. The CCHE, for example, was given a ten-fold increase in its income.

A number of specific campaigns were mounted, one such being to promote diphtheria immunisation (producing a rise in immunised children from 8 to 62 per cent within five years). After the war health education became of international concern. Reports from the World Health Organisation in 1954 and 1958 stressed that 'modern diseases arose from the very fabric of society and were inextricably linked with the life-style of individuals.[2] This challenge led to the Ministry of Health making a thorough assessment of health education needs, and the production in 1964 of the Cohen Report. Recommendations included the establishment of a strong central body to promote the development of health education on a national basis and to support all the other various agencies in their endeavours. The Health Education Council, formed in 1968, has performed this role ever since with varying success. On the local scene Health Education Officers employed by Health Authorities have rapidly expanded in number from about 50 in the mid-1960s to nearly 500 now.

THE MEDIA

Books

Books have always represented an important source of information. In a review of the opinions of people attending a GP's surgery over 15 years, Elliott-Binns[9] found that while 4.2 per cent used books as a source of advice on that occasion in 1970, twice as many turned to them in 1985. The setting up of a library in a GP's waiting room has demonstrated the popularity of books across the range of social class and educational status (many borrowers in this survey even admitting that they seldom read books, let alone used a public library).[10] Despite the enormous increase in Home Doctor books, medical dictionaries and health advice books, the evidence suggests that there is an unsatisfied demand for getting information from books (which seem not to be much used by the HEC or Health Education Officers). A non-commercial book producer is the Consumers' Association, which has been publishing its health/illness books since the first on contraception in 1963. These have been well received and have covered many of the topics which the GP's waiting room study found to be popular.

Newspapers

Newspapers find the 'human interest' story universally popular, with descriptions of individuals' experience of illness a frequent example. In 1976 the proportion of editorial space featuring such stories ranged from 13 per cent in the *Observer* to 34 per cent in the *Sun*. But how much medical information the public receive from newspapers is hard to assess. In a review of the opinions of people attending his practice over 15 years Elliott-Binns[9] found that in 1970 2.6 per cent cited newspapers as a source of advice. In 1985 the figure had risen to 3 per cent. These figures, however, are culled from one practice only.

Magazines

Undoubtedly magazines have provided more information. The corresponding figures from Elliott-Binns' study quoted above were that 5.3 per cent cited magazines as a source of advice in 1970; 5.6

per cent in 1985. A 'doctor' column or page is a regular feature in many, while others display information in a question-and-answer format which is claimed to be 'read avidly by millions'.[3]

Radio

In the early days the approach was perhaps didactic, but with Dr Charles Hill, the radio doctor, the medium achieved a remarkable intimacy and immediacy. Hill's broadcasts attracted an audience of 14 million at their peak,[1] and clearly provided a major source of knowledge for many people. More recently phone-in programmes on both local and national radio have encouraged people to seek information directly from doctors and other experts. The management of minor illness, the care of chronic conditions and perhaps more importantly, embarrassing and 'trivial' issues and questions have all been tackled. This format is clearly popular. Curiously, however, the figures from the previously quoted survey for radio are low. Perhaps its omnipresence makes its perceived influence to be underestimated, the message often being subliminal. Radio has also been the medium used in specific campaigns, most recently in the AIDS campaign.

Television

Television is undoubtedly the medium which has made the greatest impact on health education over the past ten years. The example of the Panorama programme 'Transplants — are the donors really dead?' is often cited as evidence of the power of television to present or misrepresent health information and subsequently alter people's behaviour. A sharp decline in the number of transplants followed this programme with evidence of patients dying from renal failure whose lives might otherwise have been saved. The influence of television has increased markedly in a relatively short time. Elliott-Binns' study showed that three times as many people found it a source of information in 1985 than had in 1970.

Television is the medium in which the distinction between entertainment, emotional response and education is least clear. In a recent series viewers spent many hours following the activities of a hospital. An enormous volume of health information was imparted in a minimally structured form, presented in a 'live' fashion. There were tears and laughter, operations, births and deaths, muddle and competence, bravery and cowardice. All the workings of the Health Service were seemingly laid open for inspection, enlightenment, amusement or diversion. On the other hand programmes overtly educational concerned with specific issues, such as Well Being, Food for Thought, and So You Want To Stop Smoking, have also been screened.

With almost universal ownership of video-recorders, all can be retained and replayed. The implications of all this have not yet been thought through. The public itself seems still (as with radio) not to have grasped how important a source television is: in the survey quoted, television was cited less often than books. But the rate of change suggests that a repeat survey in only a few years will show a big difference.

Medical antipathy, even paranoia, towards general health education surfaces again particularly with regard to television. An editorial in a medical journal[11] recently stated 'Unfortunately we have to live with the modern obsession that everyone has the right to know everything, but we must make sure that the BBC, the twentieth century inquisition, gets it right', a view which echoes that of J. F. South in 1857.

CONCLUSION

From its beginnings health education has contained a crusading element, and has had to contend with a reluctant medical profession guarding its knowledge. In the 100 years since 1830 the amount of information about health, illness and prevention of illness available to the general public increased steadily, and diffused slowly through the population. More recently radical changes in society have combined with the advent of radio and television to transform this situation into one in which almost every person in the 'Western' world is a target for a daily dose of persuasion. Health matters are subject to commercial, political and medical pressures — a powerful mix. Covert and overt health education is already transforming knowledge and expectations.

The general public is now on the brink of a true information explosion: this imminent Big Bang, fuelled by television and electronic and information systems' development, will give the laity such access to what was once considered 'medical knowledge' that the relationships between the roles of general public/patients/doctors will be forever altered.

REFERENCES

1. Blythe, M. (1986) A century of health education. *Health and Hygiene*, 7, 105-15
2. Coutts, L.C. and Hardy, L.K. (1985) *Teaching for health: the nurse as health educator*. Churchill Livingstone, London, p. 25
3. Williamson, J.D. and Danaher, K. (1978) *Self care in health*. Croom Helm, London
4. Anon (1854) *How to nurse sick children*. Longman, London
5. Woodham-Smith, C. (1955) *Florence Nightingale*. Penguin Books, Harmondsworth, 266
6. Nightingale, F. (1859) *Notes on Nursing*. Harrison, London
7. Slade-King, E.J. (1908) *Summary of the Reports of the Medical Officers for North Devon 1907, Exeter 1908*. Devon County Council
8. Lock, S. (1986) Self help groups: the fourth estate in medicine? *British Medical Journal*, 2, 1596
9. Elliott-Binns, C.P. (1986) An analysis of lay medicine: 15 years later. *Journal of the Royal College of General Practitioners*, 36, 542-4
10. Vanavides, C.K., Zermansky, A.G. and Pace, C. (1984) Health library for patients in general practice. *British Medical Journal*, 1, 535-7
11. Anon (Editorial) (1986) Medicine and the television. *Bristol Medico-Chirurgical Journal*, p. 125

Part 2

Present: Information Needs

6

Information for Doctors

An account of the present thinking on information needs of general practitioners, together with discussion of ways in which perception of the need may develop

Brian Higginson

INTRODUCTION

The emphasis of information technology (IT) is usually placed on the 'T'. Since the technology has far outstripped our capability to exploit it there is an increasing body of opinion that we should now concentrate on the 'I', that is, on the 'information' and the ways in which it can be handled by the technology. The technology itself can be ignored and the happy assumption made that the only limitation on our ability to get what we want out of an information system is the breadth and depth of our imagination. As the Chinese say, 'the imagination gets closer to the truth than the mind'. Developing information technology with a capital 'I' is as much an art form as a science — it requires synthesis, vision, a capability for holism or seeing the needs of the 'whole' and an understanding of human nature.

What, then, is this mysterious substance called 'information'? In the context of a microcomputer it is invisible for most of the time. Bits and bytes may be the lowest common denominator of the computer, but what are the comparable building bricks of information? A single item of data may be devoid of meaning until it is aggregated with similar items and placed in context in a defined relationship with other data. At this point it becomes information, and acquires a meaning and relevance. The graduation of data to the status of information is determined by the use to which it is being put and the function it serves. For example when data are communicated or exchanged with other data the outcome is information as part of the process of telling, informing or inferring.

If information data are shown to be reliable by being subjected to stringent scientific scrutiny they then become knowledge. For knowledge to be relevant it needs to indicate that some sort of action either should or should not be taken. Relevance is an important motivating factor in sustaining diligence in data collection, thereby improving the accuracy.

The distillation of knowledge through a process of synthesis may become wisdom, and usually comes with experience. Wisdom is necessary to avoid the mistakes which knowledgeable fools and computers make.

To make information or information systems come alive it is appropriate to draw an analogy with bricks and mortar. An architect excels in developing a feel for spatial relationships and for the many factors which affect our physical environment — light, warmth, colour, texture and noise. The systems analyst must become an information architect. This analogy can be illustrated further by visualising software which is designed to reveal information about people in a spatial context.

There are computer games which, with the aid of a 'mouse', allow the users to find their way through a two-dimensional maze. This maze can then be converted into a three-dimensional warren of passages and dead-ends which unfolds as the user walks down the corridors by manipulating the 'mouse'. These two software developments, if taken as building blocks of the imagination, may be transposed and developed in a medical context which is highly relevant to primary care.

A geographic data base will show in two dimensions the village or town in which individual general practitioners work. If an age–sex register is superimposed on that data base the patients will then appear on the map. The over-65s living alone, or the under-5s, can be made to flicker. When public domain data from the detailed household survey are added this will reveal a wealth of information about the patients living in each postcoded area. The associations between poor housing conditions and, for example, the demand on health care resources in terms of consultation rates, will become apparent.

The next step is to give a third dimension to the map so that the height of the buildings occupied by a general practitioner's patients could represent say the number of day visits made, or repeat prescriptions given, or referrals — data derived from an analysis of practice activity (see Tables 6.1 and 6.2). If a group practice looked after most of the patients in a housing estate one could then walk around the estate on the screen using the software, comparing one's own prescribing habits (and costs) with those of the other doctors in the practice. Each doctor could be hatched in a different way, or colour-coded such that the cough linctuses or tranquillisers prescribed by each individual either per thousand patients or as a gross figure would be shown.

On a larger scale if GPs agreed to merge their patient data bases which aggregated data on morbidity and mortality this would provide an invaluable treasure trove of epidemiological information. Suitably structured data could suggest where to site a nuclear power station if it was considered desirable to choose an area which has a low-density population. The data could also contribute to a scrutiny of the risks incurred by living near one. An epidemiological link between leukaemia and lymphomas could be tested by mapping patients with these diseases on a geographic data base for the United Kingdom, and then superimposing the locations of nuclear power stations on this mass of dots. Similar exercises could be undertaken when looking at occupational diseases. In this context the key which unlocks this bank vault of meaningful information is the area postcode. The fourth dimension is 'time'.

A patient who has lived the first five years of his life three miles from Sellafield, and then moved to a number of different addresses, only developing leukaemia at the age of 15 years, could then have the postcodes of all these addresses checked against those of nuclear power stations. It is at this point that the value of data on the front of the dog-eared Lloyd-George brown envelopes becomes apparent.

The power of an information system to mould and shape data according to time can yield valuable information about individual patients. The stressful events in life (the major losses and gains) such as a bereavement, losing one's job, getting married, having children, moving house and getting divorced all take on a greater depth of meaning when plotted against time. The importance of 'life charts', which consider these episodes in a psychiatric context, is becoming increasingly recognised.

In this introduction a glimpse of future possibilities has provided a backdrop against which the current information expectations of general practitioners can be described.

HISTORICAL PERSPECTIVES

There are two traditional data collection activities which started before the inception of the NHS. These are the medical record, and the information required in order to execute the administrative

Table 6.1: Suffolk Family Practitioner Committee, Practice financial profile, 1985/6

Dr Smith & Partners List size (Oct. 1985) 5629
Total population registered in Suffolk (Oct. 1985): 635,466
Total dispensing patients in Suffolk 152,595

Fee	Total payments Suffolk (£)	Total payments Practice (£)	Average/1000 patients Suffolk (£)	Average/1000 patients Practice (£)	Percentage of county average 1984/5	Percentage of county average 1985/6	Claim form	Annual usage
Temporary resident								
up to 15 days	76,238	903	123	182	134%	147%	FP 19	261
over 15 days	57,163	641	93	129	174%	140%	FP 19	261
Immediately necessary treatment	186	0.00	0.30	0.00	0%	0%	FP 106	0
Contraceptive services								
(a) Ordinary	247,913	2,044	401	412	100%	103%	FP 1001	229
(b) Intra-uterine device	41,567	658	67	133	136%	197%	FP 1002	21
Emergency treatment	21,460	330	35	67	153%	191%	FP 32	25
Night visits	122,503	1,225	198	247	108%	124%	FP 81	79
Vaccination and immunisation	310,554	2,493	503	502	92%	100%	FP 73	372
Cervical cytology	93,256	1,385	151	279	119%	185%	FP 74	210
Arrest of dental haemorrhage	106	13	0.17	2.7	0%	0%	FP 82	1
Admission of anaesthetic	22.2	0.00	0.04	0.00	0%	1,557%	FP 31	0
Maternity services	501,506	4,521	812	911	75%	112%	FP 24	68
Ancillary staff salary 70% reimbursement	1,754,227	21,746	2,761	3,863	144%	140%		
Ancillary staff — whole time equivalent (WTE)			0.69	1.22		176%		
No. of patients aged 65+					124%			
No. of patients aged 75+	441	6.87			136%	197%		
	110,990	943	175	168	94%	96%		
	48,473	394	76	70	93%	92%		
(Dispensing doctors)								
No. of prescriptions	1,073,614	33,779	7,036	6,130	90%	87%		
Prescription charges collected	340,149	14,387	317	426	126%	134%		
	(£/1,000 items dispensed)							

Table 6.2: Additional performance indicators for general practitioners

Consultations
Average time (in minutes) per consultation
Consultations per 1000 patients
Telephone consultations per 1000 patients
Day visits per 1000 patients
Night visits per 1000 patients

Referrals
Total referrals per 1000 patients
Referral as a percentage of total consultations
Percentage of urgent referrals to total referrals
Referrals as a percentage to each specialty

Investigations
Investigations per 1000 patients
Investigations as percentage of total consultations
Investigations by specialty

Prescribing details
Repeat prescriptions per 1000 patients
No. of items prescribed per quarter
Gross prescribing cost
Average no. of items prescribed per person/unit
Comparative costs for the above for the FPC, and England & Wales

No. of patients with exemption certificates (maternity, chronic sick and pre-payment)

Mortality data
Average age of death for male and female patients
Cause of death, e.g. heart/blood, cancer, respiratory, etc.

---

responsibilities of running a small business. The latter include keeping a ledger for the accountant and paying employees. The medical record may be divided into two parts — firstly the FPC registration data, that is, the name, age, sex and address. Secondly, the clinical record itself — the repository of all the information about patients which summarises their contact with outside agencies such as hospitals and the social services.

Looking through the Lloyd-George envelopes of patients who have witnessed more than 50 years of change in health care it is immediately apparent that the perception of the information needs of doctors has changed very significantly during that time. This is not necessarily a reflection on the quality of medical care received in those early years, but it is clear that the documentation of doctor-patient contacts, both in the surgery and in hospital outpatients, achieved a degree of brevity which has not been matched since. Not only have the letters from hospital doctors become much longer, but the number of investigations has increased, many of which require some further explanation in their interpretation.

The move away from what was a cottage industry in a domestic setting towards an environment which is much more organised, and has a great deal in common with a small-to-medium sized business, has made its demands on the information requirements needed to deliver the service within that changing framework. Not only do more doctors work together in groups, but their surgery premises have changed to accommodate the full primary health care team. Each new member has brought his or her own information needs. These include a message-handling system, access to the appropriate level of medical records (given that it is possible to limit access to confidential material) and a need to be kept abreast of changes in practice policies and administrative information, such as who is going on holiday and when they will be away.

There has been a significant improvement in the level of training received by the team. Vocational training for general practitioners alone has extended the length of time doctors spent in hospital by at least three years, which effectively means that a proportion of doctors spend five to six years in postgraduate training in a hospital setting, learning not only additional clinical skills but the extensive new and changing vocabulary which is associated with the specialties, with an increase in the demand for an information system which can accommodate the demands of each of these specialties.

As educational horizons widen to include more subjects in greater depth, so too does the information system needed to meet the learning requirements of those GPs who find it a necessity to keep themselves up to date in a constantly changing field. The gap between what general practitioners think they need to know — about patients, about disease and prevention, about management, about other health professions — and what it is appropriate to know if they are to remain central to the delivery of primary care is becoming increasingly obvious.

In the opening chapter of this book Ian Tait has described the basic information needs for medical records as consisting of past history, active problems, reports and letters, treatment and sensitivities (p. 11). For most practitioners it would be difficult, if not impossible, to extract such information easily and quickly from their patients' present records.

In Chapter 2 Mike Pringle points out that in only a minority of practices information is available for planning and management. Data generated within most practices are elementary. Data available from outside the practice, from the FPC, the PPA and other branches of the Health Service, are 'limited in scope and flexibility'.

In spite of the evidence of change provided by the contents of Lloyd-George envelopes the current expectations of general practitioners as to the information they need for clinical and management purposes are not high. The rest of this chapter will focus upon the ways in which they may be expected to develop.

DEVELOPING PERCEPTIONS OF NEED

The patient and his or her needs must be placed at the centre of any information system. While there are adequate opportunities to use information systems to maximise the income of either an individual doctor or a commercial interest it is an interesting commentary on UK general practice software that this is seen as a subsidiary objective to the delivery of a high standard of care. The extending circles of influence which arise from each doctor–patient contact are illustrated in Figure 6.1. Each of these added dimensions should reflect the patient's needs.

The peripheral activity of information bargaining must seem distinctly remote from the patient, but it does illustrate a growing awareness of value of information. For example some Health Authorities are helping to finance FPC computers in order to obtain the female half of their age–sex register so as to set up 'call' and 'recall' facilities for cervical cytology. General practitioners are selling prescribing data to pharmaceutical companies providing information pertinent to the development of marketing strategies. One pharmaceutical company, Ciba-Geigy, has purchased the rights to the Scottish G-Pass software which has been handed out free of charge to all GPs in Scotland who have suitable hardware. First Ciba-Geigy, and now Vamp and AAH Meditel, are acting as surrogate departmental health authorities by providing the same service to GPs in England and Wales. The proviso is that they have access to the prescribing and morbidity data from the general practitioners involved.

When information is structured there is always a danger of losing some aspect of the 'truth' which it contains while doing so. Capturing reality or 'the real world' without distortion or loss in information systems is addressed by Nigel Stott in Chapter 18, and will

Figure 6.1: Adapted from *Patient administration systems*, by Jean Roberts (Information Technology in Health Care, The Institute of Health Services Management; Kluwer Publishers)

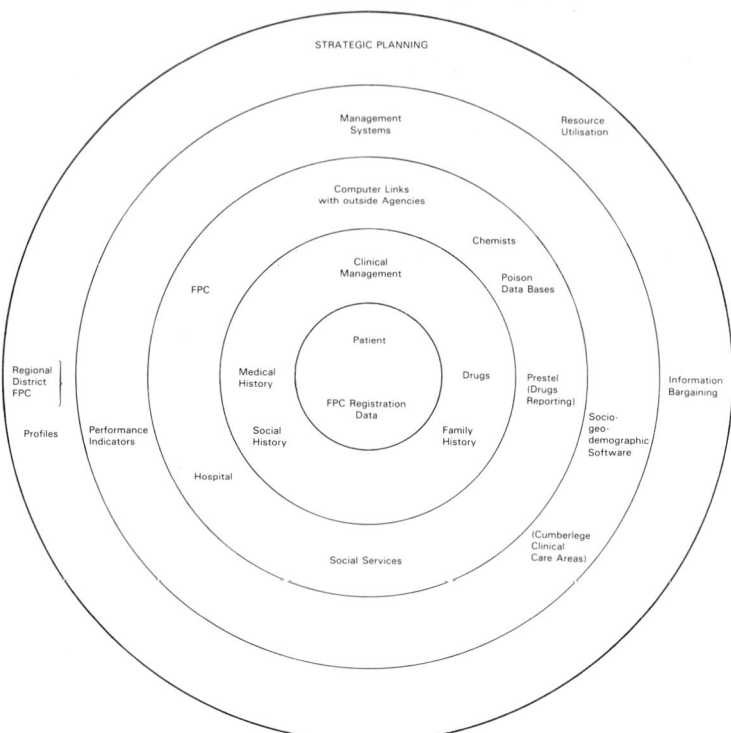

continue to exercise information specialists for many decades to come. This becomes clearer when an awareness grows of the multi-dimensional nature of some information, especially when it relates to people. While the information needs of general practitioners alone are exacting enough, if the needs of planners, administrators and commercial interests are also taken into account the pluri-potential nature of information itself becomes apparent. As practitioners become aware of the relevance of higher-quality information to their daily work, and as the vital nature of the information generated by general practice becomes more urgently realised by the rest of the health service, computers and computer networks will become essential ingredients of an information service.

Table 6.3: Generic considerations in health care information systems

Data area (function related)	Function	Problems
Resource (i.e. time and money) related data	Informed decisions Weighing options and making choices	Accuracy of decisions Integrating data from different systems
Performance indicators	Evaluation of health care delivery systems	Resistance to change
Relevance of data	Sustain motivation at point of collection	Develop data standards to check validity Housekeeping function (updating)
Data 'contours', i.e. ability to: aggregate collate transmit and distribute	Integration of data using data modelling techniques Processing of data	Agreement on definitions Adherence to these definitions at the time of collection Avoidance of epidemiological pitfalls
Access	Provide effective information service Maximise use of data via distribution network Restrict unauthorised access (maintain confidentiality)	Data protection restraints Interpretation errors

The process whereby data are collected at the point of contact between the patient and primary care and then relayed upwards to be entered at successively greater levels of aggregation, e.g. District, Region and finally DHSS, can take place so much quicker in a computerised system than in a manual system. The result can be returned to the point of collection in a matter of weeks or even days. What was in the past a strictly 'upwards' process of data collection has now developed a 'two-way' capability, with benefits to both parties.

This may be illustrated by the concept of PIs (performance indicators) which allow comparability between data collected at

Table 6.4: Information derived from a Parliamentary Answer in the House of Lords[7] (approximate average cost in 1985-6 in England)

	Total	Percentage
Total net NHS spending, current and capital per head of population	£300	
Of the above, the medical staff costs alone both in the hospital sector and the community were	£21	
Cost of general medical services was	£23	7.7%
Cost to the NHS of each GP consultation	£5.40	
Average prescription issued by GPs	£4.80	
Cost (1985/6) per week as inpatient		
Acute sector	£606	
Maternity unit	£728	
Long-stay	£321	
Geriatric	£279	
Mental illness	£270	
Mental handicap	£241	
Cost to the NHS (1984/5)* of each outpatient attendance (acute)	£21.90	
Average cost to the NHS (1984/5)* per inpatient case (acute)	£794.63	

*Data for 1985/6 not yet available.

different levels. Examples of PIs for general practice are shown in Table 6.1 and 6.2 (see also Table 6.3). This shows the quantifiable variations in activity levels in one practice over a two-year period, based on the claims for item of service work submitted. However, it could be useful to a practitioner to know the number of cervical smears carried out (per 1000 patients) within his or her immediate peer group (i.e. in a group practice), or within the locality (District Health Authority), within the Region or at national level.

The missing link throughout the current discussion about the future of primary care has been the contribution which could be made by a centrally funded information system. There are likely to be substantial savings achieved by matching activity with the level of skills available and encouraging a shift, where feasible, of care from costly sites such as hospitals to a less expensive environment in the community. Common clinical examples are the follow-up and management of diabetics and hypertensives, which can be quite easily carried out in a well-organised practice more cheaply than in hospital. The comparative costs are illustrated in Table 6.4. It has to be conceded that tangible savings only come about when outpatient staff are reduced or wards closed. Nursing shortages and financial stringencies are forcing some Health Authorities to close wards on a temporary basis during the summer months, which illustrates how this could be made a practical alternative.

The means which will enable this workload shift from hospital to primary care is to be found in information systems which contain a 'decision support module'. Expert systems with this capability are described at greater length in Chapters 11 and 12.

What is also required is a 'general practitioner information profile' which will assist GPs in their decision-making and in assessing how their work relates to agreed standards. A long-term objective could be to link information systems in such a way that health care costs can be identified per patient contact as the latter find their way through the referral system. In Chapter 20 Fitter and Garber discuss this point further.

To identify such costs requires a degree of financial data modelling which ultimately will indicate to the doctor the cost consequences of his decisions. In other words he will be able to see the justification on a cost containment basis alone of, for example, employing an extra practice nurse. If the arguments are strong enough there is reason to believe that health authorities will begin to look at ways of diverting resources to primary care in order to prevent patients having to be referred. To illustrate this point the average cost per admission to hospital is £794[1] (see Table 6.4). It follows that if a district nurse can, by her ministrations, keep 14 patients per year at home, thereby saving 14 admissions to hospital, she will pay for her salary. An estimation has been included in this calculation to include the cost of drugs, dressings, home helps and GP services.

Table 6.4 illustrates examples of the type of information which needs to be integrated into such a system. Professor Brian Jarman, who has looked at this area in some depth,[2] has developed the 'Jarman Index' for primary care which includes factors that are thought by GPs to contribute to the demand on health care resources. These include such things as 'ethnic group' and 'single parents living alone'.

The Resource Allocation Working Party (RAWP) have developed a formula for redistributing resources between Districts in order to meet the greater demands made on these in some areas, and this is currently in operation in most Regions. It is based on standardised mortality ratios (SMRs), which are considered to be a less appropriate measure of the use of health care resources than the Jarman Index, since the latter includes both morbidity and social factors which have a more direct relationship with demand.

Identification of these loci is quite a simple task using an information system based on socio-geodemographic software, as described in the introduction to this chapter.

Another development in finance planning and analysis is the use of spreadsheet software. The principle is that a table is constructed of vertical and horizontal columns of figures which bear a fixed relationship to each other, illustrating the knock-on effect on the other factors of adjusting one or more variables in either axis. This enables the user to ask 'what-if' questions. It is now possible to use spreadsheet software to examine performance in a number of areas of activity such that time and effort can be focused more sharply in order to improve performance.

The same sort of 'what-if' methodology can be applied to improving the quality of clinical care. For example, the *Risk Factors Prevalence Study* carried out by the National Heart Foundation of Australia[3] can enable a rapid calculation of the number of hypertensives who one might expect to find in a given population, indicating their likely age bands. Applying the same method in a practice will reveal the predicted incidence of patients with glaucoma and diabetes. If a morbidity index is available in the practice these calculations will give some idea of the undiagnosed patient population, and therefore the likely hit-rate if a screening drive for these treatable conditions is undertaken.

The availability and use of increasing information is opening doors for general practitioners. But managers at all levels will increasingly find themselves having to adjust to a situation in which they are not the sole custodians of the information upon which decisions are made. Politicians will find it more difficult to shelter behind the barricades of authoritative opinion when the information on which their opinion is based is subjected to scrutiny by the data providers. A pertinent example would be the process of priority ranking on an emotive issue such as taking cervical smears. Central decisions based on information generated in general practice will be exposed to judgement by general practitioners.

It seems likely that within the next few years the uptake of information technology in primary care throughout the world is going to accelerate. As in all things the question of motive is a fundamental and critical issue which has to be examined closely. Powerful vested interests in any country may foreclose the range of information options available to users, without their knowing, until the design and implementation stage of the information system is too far advanced to be changed. Unless amendments are considered and accepted in the formative stages of development of large-scale regional information systems, rewriting the programme will be expensive and may be either difficult or impractical to achieve.

In the course of describing how perceptions of need for information in general practice may develop this section has described some advances in computer technology and their implications for clinical and practice management. There is a symbiotic relationship between an awareness of what is possible, the way we think, and what we expect. Looking ahead, such increased awareness of the possible can confidently be expected to lead to increased expectations for information relating to all aspects of general practice.

WIDER ISSUES

Implications for research

New vistas open up for the use of individual patient's medical records when the implications of linking the data in all the records are considered. Each medical record may be seen as a single point of light seen from a distance on a misty night. The area illuminated is quite small. However, the accumulated glow produced by millions of small light sources is sufficient to make it possible to see a mushroom of light from some ten miles away when approaching a medium-sized town.

Data protection issues might be resolved by removing the name and address but allowing postcodes to be included. If the data item also has a code which allows it to be traced to the doctor concerned, he may then release an update. If indicated he may also seek the permission of the patient concerned. One British software company, Vamp Health, have designed their records in such a way that all the data may be collected and stored on a mainframe so that the data base is enlarging year by year. The Scottish Home and Health Department has achieved a similar result through integrating the G-Pass system with its information technology strategy.

The data in patients' notes are the primordial soup from which new species, or at least new medical knowledge of an epidemiological nature, can arise. There has not been any study of the means of acquisition of medical knowledge but some untested observations would not be out of place.

It is likely that most research work starts with a clinical 'hunch', or an idea which is later examined under more controlled conditions. There are two ways that such a hunch could be explored. Firstly, access to the large-scale data base described above on a real-time basis could allow an interaction, or mute dialogue, to be established with the data. Secondly, a message system might distribute an enquiry or hypothesis to users, who could then respond with comments or their willingness to participate in testing it out. In some cases it could be a question of asking the patient to fill in a questionnaire which can be sent electronically at low cost to multiple distribution addresses, or taken off an electronic bulletin board.

Martindale-on-Line is now available as a compact disc which is updated every year. A great deal of the information is out of date but could be retrieved from living patients with a suitable network which allowed messages to be transmitted to general practitioners in the UK, and would probably yield valid data if 50 per cent of them were linked into the network. In the long term this would reduce the need for centralised data bases.

The planning research cycle for clinical trails could be shortened and authors of medical textbooks sent enquiries about statements which may not be supported by references to scientific work. In this way assertions and clinical impressions could themselves be given life by a post-publication dialogue with the readership.

Developing an information strategy for primary care

This is an important and pressing task facing the profession. It is unlikely that the government will invest in the development of information systems for primary care until such time as a consensus has emerged with agreement on the major areas of an information strategy. This will need to address itself to some of the issues discussed in this book, and will need to find answers to the following:

(a) What information needs to be collected?
(b) How should the doctor collect this information?
(c) Who should collect this information?
(d) Does the Data Protection Act require the doctor to explain the uses to which this information can be put?
(e) Does the cost/effort involved justify collecting this information?

(f) What are the consequences of not documenting essential information, e.g. medicolegal, Inland Revenue/accountants' fees?

(g) Does the information collected lend itself to meaningful interpretation?

(h) Is there a need for linked 'information centres' to assist GPs to look after more patients in primary care?

(i) What lessons can we learn from the Japanese intensive study of the cumulative impact of technological change on the structure of society — the so-called 'wired society'?

(j) Has any attempt been made to examine the needs of general practice software industry?

(k) Are the aims of the Department of Trade and Industry, viz. 'to provide a framework or climate in which business can prosper' (Geoffrey Pattie, former Minister for Information Technology[4]), compatible with the cost containment objectives of the DHSS?

While these questions may seem academic to most general practitioners there are those who see the need for all who work in primary care to have at their disposal what is described as a 'distance independent communications environment' which allows them to communicate with colleagues and agencies from any location within the practice. This must lead eventually to a system which is similar to cellular radio, is fully mobile and is linked to portable end-user terminals. There is now a persuasive argument to utilise the information-carrying capabilities of 'intelligent cards' as part of an integrated information system which takes advantage of the willing co-operation of patients as custodians of their own files. The difficulty of communicating with colleagues in the primary health care team who have to cover a wide geographical 'patch' can be largely overcome by using an integrated system. If used to its fullest advantage it must make a significant contribution to the working of the team. There are probably few other areas of activity which can make use of a system to such good effect with all the capabilities which have been described.

IN CONCLUSION

The observant reader will have noticed that this chapter, which looks

Figure 6.2

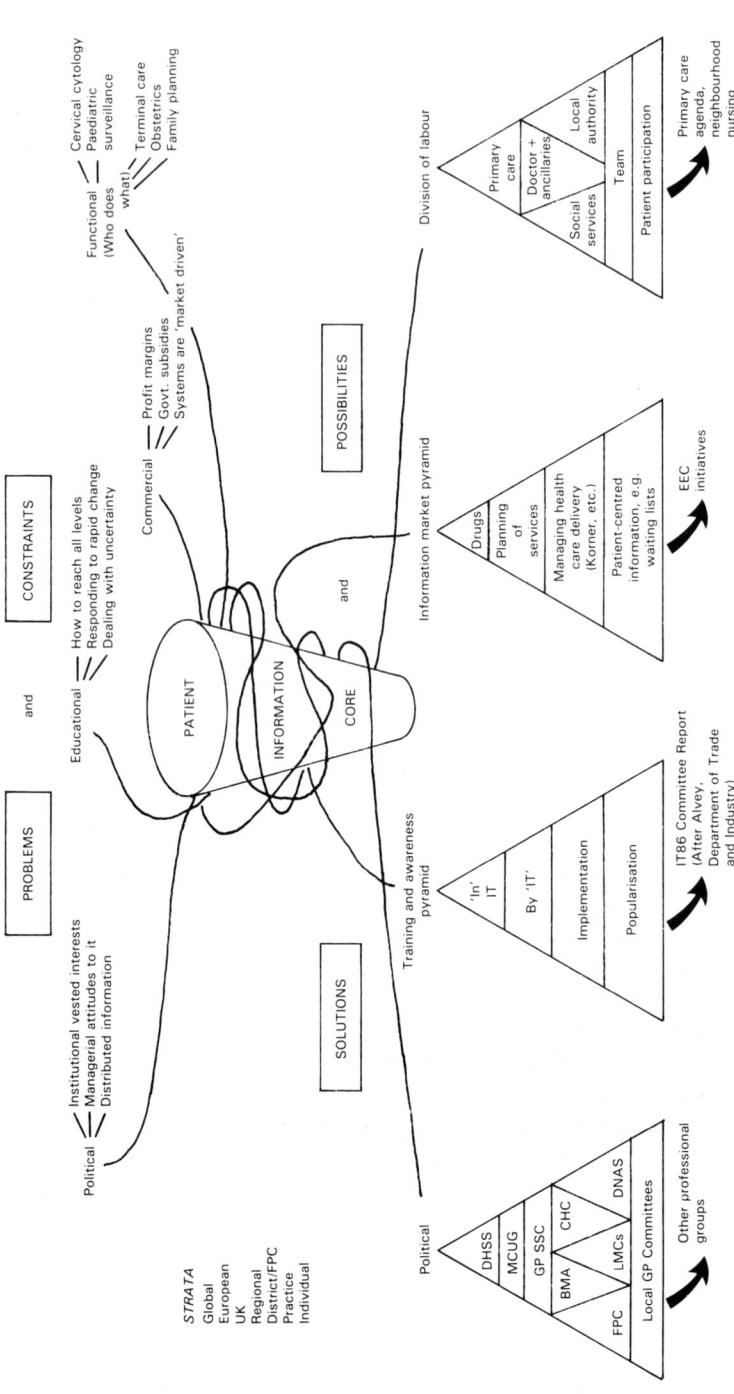

at the information requirements of general practitioners, has overlapped with many of the subject headings of other chapters in the book. In information system terms these areas of overlap are described as 'hooks' which allow the information in the different parts of the system to be satisfactorily linked together. Some aspects of these 'hooks' are touched on in Table 6.3, and some of their interrelationships illustrated in Figure 6.2.

If these 'hooks' are identified before computerised information systems are written, the extra cost of programming them into the system is minimal. If they are either not identified or ignored, then the cost consequences of rewriting programs may be prohibitive and perhaps impractical. There is therefore a strong argument for some central initiative to stimulate debate on this crucial issue. There is a need for a common basic specification for primary care.

Ultimately we will have to reach a compromise between the desirable, the feasible and the affordable. However, much more is at stake than is generally appreciated, and very little attention has been given to the consequences of allowing unco-ordinated development of information systems for primary care south of the Scottish border, although some warning shots have been fired by the Arthur Andersen report.[5] There has been little evidence that heed has been paid to this excellent report, which is mandatory reading for those who are interested in GP computing. However, there are grounds for optimism. The House of Commons Select Committee has now published a report[6] recommending that computers in general practice should be funded.

The next five to six years are going to be viewed by historians as one of the most important half-decades in the development of primary care in the UK. At the end of this period the present slowly growing expectations of general practitioners concerning their information needs will be seen as the first faltering steps into a new world.

ACKNOWLEDGEMENT

I am grateful to Dr Geoffrey Rivett, Senior Principal Medical Officer at the DHSS, and Mr Gerry Gold in the Corporate Data Administration, for their helpful comments on the original draft. I am also indebted to Mrs Jean Roberts for permission to adapt Figure 6.1 from an article published by Kluwer, and to both Mr Robinson of Suffolk FPC and Mr Tallis of Barnsley FPC for their help in providing data and documents on performance indicators for general practitioners.

REFERENCES

1. *Health and Personal Social Service Statistics for England* (1986) Table 2.6, p. 19
2. Jarman, B. (1983) Identification of underpriviledged areas. *British Medical Journal*, 286, 1705-9
3. National Heart Foundation of Australia (1983) *Risk Factor Prevalence Study*
4. Pattie, G. (1987) Backsliding in the boardroom. Minister for Information Technology urges industry to grasp the opportunities for technological progress. *The Times*, 11 March
5. Arthur Andersen & Co. (1985) *Report of a study of family practitioner services administration and the use of computers*. DHSS Welsh Office
6. Social Services Committee (1987) *First report from the social services committee 1986-87: primary health care*, vol. 1. HMSO, London
7. *Hansard*, House of Lords, 9 March 1987, No. 1356, Column 924

7

Information for People

Joan Mant and Richard Westcott

Like other fascinating phrases this one, 'information for people', is capable of many interpretations, so we should make clear the meaning we propose to use. 'Information' is described by the dictionary as 'imparted knowledge of fact'; we shall define 'people' as those registered with a doctor, whether 'patients' or not. So we shall be looking at knowledge needed by a population which might at some time need the services of the primary care team.

Who decides what information these people need? More and more that decision is being taken by the consumers themselves, their interest and awareness fed by newspapers, TV, and increasingly reports from the medical profession and the DHSS among others.

In one year 40,000 people wrote to the 'agony aunt' Claire Rayner asking for help.[1] She classified their requests into nine categories according to the type of information needed.

(1) about anatomy and physiology;
(2) anxieties about pregnancy and childbirth;
(3) birth control problems;
(4) problems with child care, especially feeding, sleep, skin care, potty training and immunisation;
(5) mental health;
(6) sexual problems;
(7) about plastic surgery;
(8) about particular illnesses;
(9) about problems of the old.

Forty thousand people seeking information about personal health and illness from one journalist in one year provides an idea of the scale of unmet need.

Besides health, illness and treatment people increasingly seek information about how to choose a general practitioner or practice, what services are offered and how to use the health services. At the boundary between people and patients, patient participation groups, each based on a practice, have become more common. With their main activities being health education, community care and feedback about the services in the practice such groups both demonstrate their need for information and provide a practical method of obtaining it by their own activities and pressure.

AVAILABLE SERVICES

The first fact which most people need to know is where their local practice may be, and whether they have a choice to exercise.

Which practice?

It is true that most of us still inherit our family doctors (like silver teaspoons) and on moving to another district ask a neighbour for guidance. A Scottish study showed well over half of respondents had chosen their doctors this way. For those who do not, what information is available? Where are the directories, are they kept up to date, do they contain the information that a busy Mum with toddlers needs?

Having discovered the practices which are within walking distance, or on an easy bus route, the next questions are what are they like, what services do they offer and how do they work? Unless the practices produce a leaflet or brochure this information is often hard to come by. It is interesting that it has taken so long for general practitioners to realise that people need information *before* committing themselves, in order to be able to make a choice which is sensible for them, as well as *after* registering with a practice in order to discover how it is organised.

How is it organised?

Unless both patients and doctors understand the way the practice is organised and the rules of the game, resentment and inefficiency abound. Practice leaflets are an opportunity to inform new patients (and remind old ones) what surgeries are available and when, of arrangements for home visits, emergencies and out-of-hours calls, of preventive and other services which are available and how to obtain them. For people as patients these are basic information needs.

Primary care services

In practice booklets, where they exist, a note is usually made of members of the primary care team who are attached to the practice. This may well be the only way in which the names of nurses, health visitors and social workers who work in the community are made known to the people among whom they work. The need for information about who to contact and how to contact them for nursing services, for social services, for meals on wheels, home helps and allowances is expressed by lay people, but rarely acknowledged by local authorities or health authorities. Information about local pharmaceutical services is equally rare. Edwards[2] points out that local pharmacists run the biggest well-person clinics in the community, yet there is virtually no information available to the public on how to use this potentially very useful health professional.

Hospital services

Judging by the number of references to use and misuse of hospital services there would seem to be a clear need for people to be informed as to the appropriate use of these services. With open access to casualty departments, accident and emergency services and other specialised clinics the need for information guiding people to appropriate use of these hospital-based services is apparent.

Voluntary services

These exist to satisfy a need. People have needs which can be helped by voluntary services. Unfortunately the dichotomy between health professionals and volunteers often extends to the professionals being unaware of the excellent resources that voluntary organisations can offer, both in their own localities and nationally. Moreover it is commonplace to find that the lay public, as well as professionals, are ignorant as to how voluntary organisations can be contacted.

USING THE SERVICES

Another basic information need is to help people decide when to use what service, or indeed any service at all. The extent to which people should treat their own minor illnesses is a matter for continuing debate. What *is* known is that people frequently seek advice for minor self-limiting illness, but treat themselves for symptoms which are potentially serious.[3] The need for people to be given advice to help them distinguish between these two categories is clear. That such advice would be welcome and effective was shown by the results following the production of a booklet by the Health Education Council *Treating yourself*.[4] A survey showed that 70 per cent of its readers said that a visit to the doctor had been saved.[1]

Another publication, *Minor illness: how to treat it at home*,[5] also resulted in 'considerably more health care and visits to the general practitioner'. Follow-up of these surveys showed that 'what patients need to respond appropriately to common symptoms of illness is a simple reference manual rather than an educational programme'.[1]

HEALTH AND DISEASE

Regarding the enquiries about illness addressed to her, Claire Rayner commented:

> 'Far too many readers ask me to explain to them what their doctor meant when he said they had high blood pressure, low blood pressure, angina, fibroids, ovarian cyst . . ., the list is long. Even more distressing are those who write and say the doctor has diagnosed diabetes, cholecystitis, spastic colon or whatever, and had told them to follow a particular diet and will I please provide the diet?'[1]

These enquiries reflect the unmet needs of patients for specific information. The experience of BACUP[6] shows that similar needs exist among many patients with cancer. And not only patients with cancer. Among the enquirers are numbered the families and friends of people with cancer. The ripples widen. Neighbours help to care for old people who are incontinent or have had strokes, and need to understand what is happening and how best to help. Illness affects many people beside the patient. These people also have information needs.

The relevance of health information, for maintaining health and preventing illness, is as yet not universally appreciated by the general public. Pressure has tended to arise from without rather than within. In 1976 the DHSS report, *Prevention and health: everybody's business*, placed the responsibility for his own health on each individual.[7] In 1980 the American Surgeon-General declared 'You the individual can do more for your own health and well-being than any doctor, any hospital, any drugs, and exotic medical service'.[1] Yet there is evidence, from jogging to health food shops, to show that interest in ways of maintaining health and preventing illness is steadily increasing. The College of Health recognised this need for information at its foundation in 1983 — 'So the main purpose of the new College is the same as that of the other [Royal Medical] Colleges, that is to improve education, in our case the education of lay people'.[8]

TREATMENT AND MANAGEMENT

When someone has been diagnosed as having a complaint such as diabetes there are a number of things which they need to know about their management and treatment. Often, however, they are at a great disadvantage unless they happen to have personal experience through a relative or friend of what to expect. In a survey among diabetic patients reported by Gann,[1] 80 per cent failed to administer their insulin properly, 50 per cent tested their urine in a way which would distort the results and 75 per cent had unacceptable meals with unacceptable spacing. Many of these patients clearly were not aware of their need for information. Similarly in a survey into communication in a coronary care unit 80 per cent of the patients interviewed expressed an interest in learning about their treatment, only 40 per cent reported having been told. With prescribing the same situation is commonplace. Patients not only need to know how often and when to take the drugs they have been prescribed; they also need to be warned of potential problems such as interactions with particular foods and drinks or possible side-effects. In another survey recently,[9] while over 90 per cent of patients had been told how to take their drugs only 32 per cent had been informed verbally about side-effects, with only 14 per cent receiving written information. A final twist is that although over 90 per cent had been told how to take their drugs, at present up to half of all patients do not take their drugs as prescribed.[9]

The situation regarding information for treatment and management appears to be that frequently both doctors and patients are unaware of what the patient needs to know but doesn't — and that when doctors attempt to educate people it is often in terms the patient either does not understand or does not remember.

THE FUTURE

How may the information needs of patients and the public at large be expected to develop? This review has shown there to be a widespread feeling among health authorities and organisations that more information should be available: about how to choose a service, how to use the service and about health illness management and treatment. The Declaration of Alma Ata states as its fourth point that 'the people have a right and a duty to participate individually and collectively in the planning and implementation of their health care'. The World Health Organisation pronounced in 1983 that 'health sciences and technology have come to a point where their further contribution to health standards can make a real impact only if the people themselves become full partners in health protection and promotion'.

Yet for the most part people in general are only just beginning to appreciate that they have these needs and, more important, that they are allowed to voice them. Developments in society at large have led to an erosion of professional monopolies. Increasing democratisation involves sharing information as well as power. The common criticism of doctors that they fail to give adequate information[10] is being overtaken by the positive conviction that people should become active partners in management and prevention in sickness and health.

Both the need to know, and the vigour with which this knowledge is pursued, will undoubtedly increase.

REFERENCES

1. Gann, R. (1986) *The health information handbook.* Gower, Aldershot
2. Edwards, C. (1987) The pharmacist in primary care. *Update,* 15 January, p. 134
3. Jones, R.V.H. (1976) Self-medication in a small community. *Journal of the Royal College of General Practitioners, 26,* 410–13
4. Health Education Council (1976) *Treating yourself.* HEC, London
5. Health Education Council (1984). *Minor illness: how to treat it at home.* HEC, London
6. British Association of Cancer Patients (1987) *Breaking the silence on cancer; a review of 1986.* BACUP, London
7. Department of Health and Social Security (1976) *Prevention and health: everybody's business.* HMSO, London
8. Young, M. (1983). The four purposes and six methods. *Self Health, 1,* 3–4
9. McMahon, T., Clark, C.M. and Bailie, G.R. (1987) Who provides patients with drug information? *British Medical Journal, 294,* 355
10. Fletcher, C.M. (1973) *Communication in medicine.* Nuffield Provincial Hospital Trust, London

Part 3
What Technology Offers Now

8
What Microcomputers Offer Doctors Now

Stewart Reid and Bob Jones

By the end of this chapter the reader should have a clear idea of what computer systems can offer general practitioners in 1987. The major applications will be discussed under four headings: Finance, Organisation, Medical Records and Audit. None will be covered in detail as this varies from country to country, but principles will be outlined.

FINANCE

Financial applications have formed the basis of computerisation in most countries other than the UK.

Patient billing

In countries where patients pay at the time of consultation there are very few computerised practices who do not use a computerised billing system. Once a 'bill' is entered on to the computer it can be accessed easily and rapidly in response to account status enquiries; it can be printed at any time of the month at will; it can be automatically dated and aged. Account summaries (for example for all accounts which are three months outstanding) can be generated. For all practical purposes accounts are never lost, so the only source of inaccuracy is the original entry. Provided a clear system of entry is established and followed by all staff, patient billing is accurate and prompt.

A further refinement is instant billing. Under this system all patients are presented with a computer-generated account at the end of the consultation. This account may be paid and receipted immediately, and proponents claim that with instant billing the percentage of payments made at the time of consultation increases. Fewer bills generated in this way are queried, and unless the account ages more than a month no postage is involved.

Billing systems are pretty standard, whether in banking, retailing or the provision of services. Many 'packaged' billing systems are available.

Practical finance management

Spreadsheet programs which enable the practice finances to be monitored effectively are readily available in Australia, New Zealand and the USA. They work as follows. Each expenditure item (such as salaries, drugs and dressings, postage) and each income item (e.g. patient fees, government subsidy) is assigned a code. The code is noted when each cheque is written and each deposit made. When the bank statement is received each item on the statement is marked with the appropriate code. From this coded statement the amounts of money spent and received are entered on the computer. The totals displayed on the computer screen can be checked after entry against the bank statement. A monthly report can be generated together with a monthly running report for comparison to the figures of the previous year (Table 8.1).

Table 8.1: Financial management report (£)

	April	May	June	Year to date	Total last year	Annual budget
Salaries	10,000	10,400	10,500	30,900	110,000	130,000
Drugs/dispensing	1,000	—	2,000	3,000	9,000	12,000
Postage, etc.	200	—	200	650	2,000	2,300
Patient fees	8,000	10,000	9,500	27,500	95,000	110,000
Government subsidy, etc.	4,500	5,000	4,750	13,750	60,000	72,000

This mechanism permits very tight financial control of the practice and is of great assistance in budgeting. In Britain one such financial package tailored to the needs of practitioners working in the National Health Services has recently become available.

ORGANISATION

The purpose of general practice is to provide primary health care for all people. As in other occupations and businesses in order to fulfil this purpose a number of separate activities are involved which have to be organised, controlled and co-ordinated. For some of these activities computer programs are not available. For others, such as appointment systems, they are rare in some countries, commonplace in others. Effective programs are, however, widely available for a number of aspects of practice organisation. In practices which have microcomputers these programs have largely superseded the manual systems previously in use.

Patient registration

Whereas finance is the most commonly used function in Australia, New Zealand and the USA, in the UK the patient register is the basis of all major functions.[1] Up to 20 facts are usually entered as basic information about each person on the register. These include names, age (date of birth), sex, marital status, address, telephone number, date registered, date records received. This register can be regarded either as the basis of the medical record of each patient or as the primary management tool. It is used for both purposes. The numbers of people registered with the practice, the changes which occur over time, the proportion of the practice population, male and female, in different age groups can be made available for continuing review. In most computer systems analyses are available either according to individual factors or to combinations of factors chosen by the practice.

Patient call and recall

This is a very important computer application in general practice and one appreciated by patients.[2] The principles of call and recall are to

(a) define the patient population at risk;
(b) define the conditions requiring recall, and the frequency of recall;
(c) record those patients in whom 'episodic action' is taken;

(d) identify the remainder — those who have missed out — and devote the major effort to them.

(a) Population at risk

This depends first and foremost on being able to define the practice population. It is necessary to have a definition of 'who is a patient'. In Britain, with long-established official patient registration, this is not a problem. In other countries individual practices or the profession collectively may have to establish a definition for themselves. In New Zealand the Royal New Zealand College of General Practitioners has, for example, formulated a definition of a 'practice patient' specifically to permit patient recall without overstepping the boundary of professional behaviour. In New Zealand practice patients are defined as 'a patient who receives services from the practice or who has indicated his or her intention to attend the practice for medical services, and who belongs to a family one member of which has received services within the last two years'. So, for example, for childhood immunisations the population at risk would be all children under a specified age from families who fell under the definition of 'practice patients' as quoted. With a computer it is easy to ensure that all children who should be on the immunisation recall system are indeed on it, a task which can be tedious when performed manually.

(b) Conditions for call and recall

For children the commonest reason for inviting them to attend the practice is for a primary course of immunisation. For adults it may be policy to recall patients for blood pressure checks, to teach breast examination, to check Rubella status, to give influenza vaccine to those at risk. It may be advantageous to combine appropriate preventive activities in one appointment.

In most systems it is possible to specify parameters for call and recall, e.g. to call all women aged 35–40 years who have never had a cervical smear, to recall all children aged five years who have received their primary immunisations but not a preschool booster.

These parameters may be fixed, or may be chosen by the practice.

(c) Episodic prevention

In practices with a policy of encouraging preventive procedures doctors are increasingly carrying out 'opportunistic health promotion',[3] i.e. checking up on aspects of health status when the patient consults for something else.

Such episodic prevention (which must be entered on the computer record otherwise it will sabotage the accuracy of the recall system) is encouraged in some systems by the existence of a 'health care screen' which can be viewed during the consultation or printed out as a card. The date of the last BP recording, cervical smear or tetanus immunisation can be checked. In one general practice computer package in New Zealand such a 'screening template' is an integral part of the system and one of its most effectively used applications.

For practices in which major emphasis is laid on opportunistic health promotion most of the population at risk will have been seen in the course of normal consultations and their health status should have been checked. The relatively few people who have escaped this net are the defaulters who need special invitations.

In other practices, particularly in the UK, it is assumed that opportunistic health promotion will 'catch' only a minority of the population at risk. In this case the 'defaulters' comprise all patients at risk unless proved otherwise.

(d) The defaulters

For those people who need invitations to attend the practice computer systems offer a number of options. Sticky labels can be produced, printed with names and addresses. Individualised letters for each preventive or surveillance activity can be designed and printed out by the computer. Lists of patients can be produced, who may be telephoned, visited or sent a card.

Drugs and prescribing

The ability to print prescriptions, both one-off and on a repeat basis, is a function provided by most general practice computer systems. In the UK it is the function which after registration is the most frequently used and appreciated.[4] Early in development the British Government agreed to provide computer stationery for prescriptions. The prescription pad issued for use in the National Health Service measures 7 × 4¼ inches. The computer stationery originally designed to fit a small printer measures 7 × 8½ inches including a detachable portion. The extra space has been used to provide a tear-off strip alongside the prescription form (Figure 8.1). The information and messages which can be printed on this slip vary

Figure 8.1

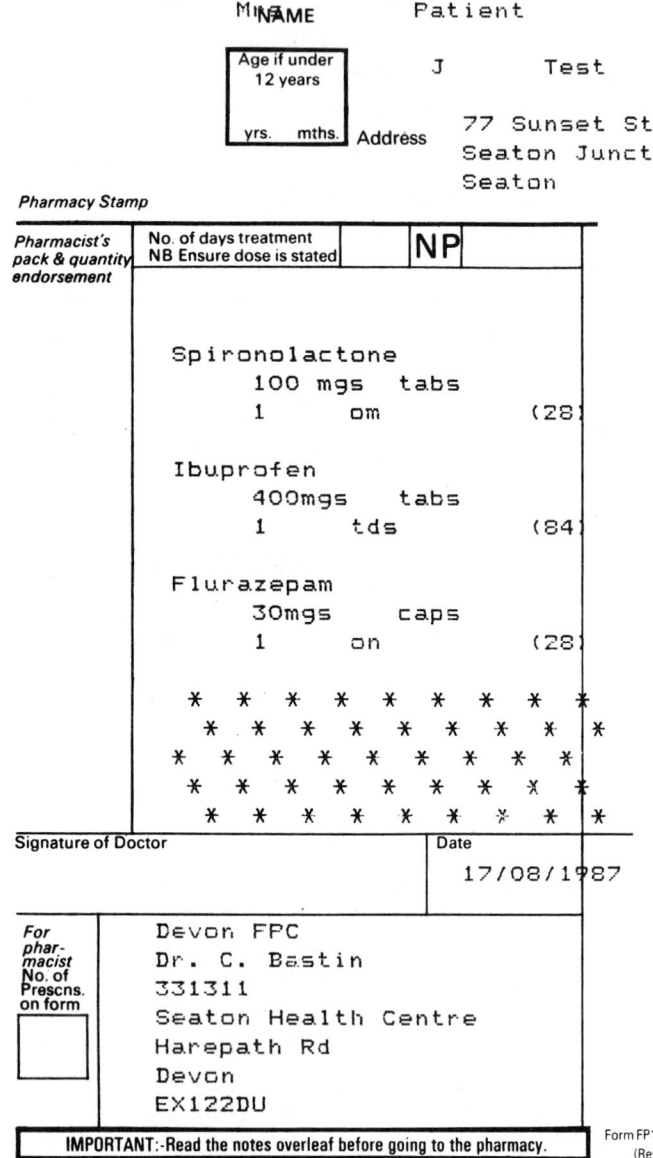

Pricing Office use only

Mrs J Patient
77 Sunset Strip
Seaton Junction
Seaton
Devon

REPEAT MEDICATION. The following drugs are currently being issued. Please indicate drugs required and bring to Health Centre. PLEASE ALLOW 48HRS NOTICE FOR RENEWAL.

    1 Spironolactone 100 mgs 1 om
Pse see Doctor for next repeat
    2 Ibuprofen 400mgs 1 tds
        11X More
    3 Flurazepam 30mgs 1 on
        23X More
    4 BURINEX K 1 om
        6X More
    9 Septrin Allergy

   10 MFV JECT 1amp

Please show this slip to any DOCTOR or HOSPITAL whenever you are treated.
Reference 10000 17/08/1987

with the system. They can usually be altered at the discretion of the practice to include not only factual information for the pharmacist, patient or practitioner but also messages such as 'Happy Christmas', or notice of practice arrangements during a Bank Holiday.

One-off prescribing

Using computer stationery in the printer a one-off prescription can either be made out from prescribing data already stored about the patient concerned or keyed in afresh. In practices where the computer is an office tool this facility is used only occasionally. In a few practices where there is a terminal in the consulting room it is used routinely.

Repeat prescribing

The issue of prescriptions to patients on a routine basis without direct doctor–patient contact has over the past ten years become commonplace in UK general practice. Factors encouraging this habit include an increasingly elderly population who need regular medication for chronic conditions, with surveillance intervals ranging from three months to one year, as opposed to the advice of the DHSS to issue a prescription for no more than one month's supply.

The standard procedure is that for each patient who needs regular medication a drug record is raised on the computer. This record specifies the name, formulation and dose of each drug, the number of drugs to be issued, the interval between issues, the instructions for the patient, and the number of prescriptions authorised before review (Figure 8.2). When a repeat prescription is requested the drug record for that patient is shown on the screen, the request checked, the drug selected and the prescription printed. Printing can be done individually or in batches. In some systems the facility to pre-print prescriptions for issue on a nominated date is provided.

Safety

Most programs for prescribing contain simple safety features which operate automatically. All prescriptions requested have to be checked as authorised before they can be printed. The number of

Figure 8.2: Example of a repeat prescription record for a patient

REPEAT DRUG/REGIME	FIRST GIVEN	LAST ISSUE	AUTH	ISSUED	QTY	Pres/GP	DAYS	LAT.	NEXT DUE
Brinaldix K 1 OD	02/03/84	19/06/87	20	14	60	TABS DR. R. JONES	60	7	18/07/87
Gaviscon 1 PRN	02/03/84	19/05/87	6	5	30	SACHETS DR. R. JONES	30	7	18/06/87
Nitrazepam 1 ON	02/03/84	06/05/87	31	32	30	TABS 5mg DR. R. JONES	30	7	FINISHED
Ibuprofen tablets 1 OM	18/09/85	19/05/87	10	10	60	TABS 200mg DR. R. JONES	0	0	FINISHED

times a prescription may be issued without reauthorisation is shown on the screen, and the number of times previously issued is also shown on the screen and often printed on the side-slip. In more sophisticated systems when a new item is added to a patient's drug list contraindications to its use and possible side-effects are displayed. In addition possible interaction with drugs which the patient is already having can be shown together with a list of drugs to which the patient has been allergic in the past.

Audit of computer prescribing by individual practitioners, and by a partnership as a whole, can be provided by most general practice systems. Clearly if a general practitioner writes his one-off prescriptions manually, and uses a computer for his repeat prescribing, it is only his repeat prescribing behaviour which the computer can analyse.

Most systems can also identify those patients who are on a particular drug, such as digoxin or indomethacin. This may be useful either to review therapy in a cohort of patients with the same complaint, or to be able to take action if a drug proves to have a severe previously unrecognised side-effect.

MEDICAL RECORDS

The advent of computers is one of the factors which have increased the need to analyse medical records and their function. Manual records traditionally have consisted of identification details, a record of consultations on a continuing basis, and reports from hospitals and laboratories. More recently summary cards, cards for preventive procedures and protocols for specific diseases have been added.

Computerised records, on the other hand, while based on identifiable individuals, have developed by adding summary information and drug information to identification details of patients. It is only the sophisticated (by present standards) general practitioner systems which cater for storage of results of investigations of hospital reports and a record of consultations on a continuing basis. The options available for computerised medical records are summarised in Table 8.2.

In the majority of general practitioner systems the medical record of a patient consists of identification details of each 'registered' patient, the drug treatment which each patient is having on a regular basis, priority details such as allergies or drug sensitivities,

Table 8.2: Stages in computerisation of medical records

On computer

A. Patient register
   Demographic details — + Paper record

B. A. Plus
   Personal risk/priority details
   Summary of —
     immunisation — + Paper record
     chronic disease
     regular drug therapy

C. A. Plus B. Plus
   Medical record summary
   Family history — + Paper record
   Social history
   Preventive care information
   Current drug therapy
   Current problem list

D. A. Plus B. Plus C. Plus
   Continuation notes
   Specialist letters
   Results of investigations

information concerned with preventive procedures which are appropriate for that patient and a list of major diagnoses from which the patient suffers. It is notable that the basis of all manual records is a chronological account of consultations, whereas this facility is only available on a very few computer systems. All but a tiny minority of computerised practices at present continue to use manual paper records as the main medical record — with the computer record frequently being used as a summary sheet.

Further factors which discourage the use of computers for the routine recording of medical data about individual patients are the rigidity of the computer record compared to the many different ways in which a paper record can be used, the fact that writing and drawing are easier for most practitioners than typing, and the lightness and convenience of a paper record compared to the immobility of most computer systems.

FEEDBACK AND AUDIT

The importance of feedback of information about how well or badly a practice is doing, compared to what it would like to do or thinks it is doing, is now recognised more widely than a decade ago. Analyses of methods used successfully in business[5] and in education[6] have converged to show that the setting of objectives and the presence of feedback to find out whether the objectives are being met are essential for successful management, whether it be of an office, a sales force or a practice.

This is an area where current general practice computer systems score heavily over manual systems. With a manual system it is possible using an age–sex register with tagging and multiple entries to produce a list of girls who have not been immunised against Rubella. It is possible to identify those patients with asthma, with thyroid disease or with hypertension, and to work through their manual records to discover whether they have been regularly monitored or whether they have slipped through the net. It is possible to identify elderly people living alone who have not been seen in the past year. But with each additional survey undertaken the amount of checking and paper increases, record envelopes bulge with special cards, and they split. In some practices without a computer processing the information collected, analysing this information and producing useful feedback has become a major occupation — expensive and arguably self-defeating.

On the other hand, the ability to identify individuals with shared characteristics is a basic facility of most computer systems. It is the foundation of call-and-recall as described earlier in this chapter. Moreover, provided entries are made when a test is done or examination carried out, it is possible to identify easily those patients whose clinical management may have been faulty — such as a patient with thyroid disease who has not had a T4 estimation within a specified time, or patients being treated for hypertension who have not had their pressures taken for a long time. If a practitioner or practice has policies concerning clinical care, provided the relevant facts are entered on the computer record it is easy to discover how well the policies are being carried out. Feedback is easily and rapidly available. Feedback about practice statistics based on registration details is also available on almost all systems — and can be used for planning. For example information about an increase or decrease in the number of males and females registered with the practice, and the age groups in which the changes occur, is important when a practice is planning new services or modifying those already in operation.

For practices with computerised appointment systems feedback about delays, waiting times and non-attenders is possible. In general the ability to provide feedback information for use in audit is one of the stronger points of current general practitioner computer systems.

OTHER FUNCTIONS

There are some subsidiary functions which are available in a number of general practice systems.

Word processing

Although most systems have the facility for printing sticky labels and producing standard letters it is becoming more common for true word processing to be offered as part of a package. The main use for word processing in practice is for writing referral letters, recording the minutes of meetings or writing reports and scientific articles. Patient information leaflets can also be stored and produced when required.

Information systems

Most readers will be aware of Videotex and Teletext information systems, examples being Prestel in the UK and Viatel in Australia. Access by the practice computer to some large external data bases is also possible. There are data bases providing information about drugs, poisons and prescribed drugs taken in overdose. There are others (e.g. Medline) which provide references to journals, books, abstracts and other medical publications. Although the amount of information available to general practitioners is currently not great, it is clear that this is an area overdue for expansion. An account of medical data bases and developments in the pipeline can be found in Chapter 10.

In addition to accessing external information systems use can be made of a practice computer to build up a personal bibliography in which articles and abstracts can be stored. This necessitates construction of an indexing system, preferably with multiple keyword access.

Education and research

Because information about individual patients is stored in most practice computers, and because functions are available to identify groups of people with common characteristics, the opportunity to undertake research or to use the facts for educational purposes is obvious. It is important to understand that the mere possession of a computer will not turn a practitioner into a medical researcher, but the ready availability of relevant information is a big advantage. The computer may be the tool which brings research within reach.

CONCLUSION

As this review has shown, the most important computer applications in general practice at present relate to practice finance, preventive health care, prescribing and medical records. At several points it has been suggested that there is a long way to go before computer systems offer enough flexibility, ease of use and portability to meet the presently conceived information needs of practitioners in their daily work. What computer systems do offer now is an efficient method of performing certain office functions, a greatly increased ability for feedback and audit, and opportunities for education and research.

In addition, and this should not be underestimated when considering what computers offer family doctors, introduction of a computer system into a practice leads to consideration of working methods and a review of practice procedures.

Systematic review, essential to good management, is rare in general practice. A computer system can be a catalyst for change in those practices which accept the challenge.

REFERENCES

1. Department of Health and Social Security (1985) *General practice computing: evaluation of the micros for GPs scheme*. Final Report. HMSO, London
2. Reid, J.S. (1984) How to improve anticipatory care using a computer. *New Zealand Family Practitioner*, 97, 688–9
3. Stott, N.C.H. and Davis, R.H. (1979) The exceptional potential in each primary care consultation. *Journal of the Royal College of General Practitioners*, 29, 201–5

4. Fitter, M.J., Garber, J.R., Herzmark, G.A., Robinson, D. and Jones, R.V.H. (1986) *A prescription for change*. HMSO, London

5. Drucker, P.F. (1968) *The practice of management*. Pan Books in association with William Heinemann, London

6. Pereira Gray, D.J. (1979) *A system of training for general practice*, 2nd edn. Occasional Paper 4. Royal College of General Practitioners, London

9

What Computers and Broadcasting Offer Patients

John Chisholm

COMPUTERS

Computers have the potential to facilitate improved patient care. However, by far the greater part of present experience with computers in medicine has been obtained when the computer is operated by doctors or other health care professionals. Situations in which the patient uses the computer are still comparatively rare.

Within British general practice, Dove has written of his findings when 60 young women had their medical and social history taken by a computer before having an interview with the doctor.[1] It seemed that the computer-patient interview had therapeutic benefits, enabled the doctor to communicate more quickly and in greater depth in the time available, and in effect magnified the time which the doctor could spend with the patient. The therapeutic benefits particularly derived from the nature of the computer's interrogation — 'the computer is never tired, and it can be programmed to give a sense of infinite patience' — and the sensitive indication of those areas about which the patient was most concerned. Certainly most patients found the method acceptable.

However, inasmuch as the average length of the automated interview is 90 minutes, these methods cannot readily be extended into routine general practice with its average consultation time of five or six minutes, although they would perhaps have benefits when a patient first registers with a practice, or presents with a difficult psychosocial problem.

Dove regards such computer-interviewing techniques as 'a logical extension of the process of computer diagnosis'. A more common development within the medical environment has been the use of computer-assisted learning — almost the reverse situation, in which the patient learns from the computer, rather than the computer receiving information from the patient.

Computer-assisted learning

Computer-assisted learning (CAL) has certain clear advantages over alternative techniques such as learning from the printed page or from a teacher. It provides a consistent quality of instruction that does not vary by teacher or over time. It does not tire. The computer may be more readily available than a teacher. Lessons on a computer can be updated with ease. The computer can objectively monitor and report on the progress of the student.[2] Perhaps most importantly the computer gives control of the lesson to the patient, who has the option of choosing and exploring what he wants or needs to learn, and repeating material when necessary.[3] The computer may be particularly appropriate for instruction in potentially embarrassing topics.[4] Some believe the educational strategies of self-pacing and interaction are particularly effective in teaching, and describe these as the fortes of computer-based education.

A classification of CAL into four categories has been suggested: tutorial dialogue, computational aid, simulation and modelling, and the discipline of programming. Tutorials allow scope for student interaction, and can include very basic drill-practice routines, multiple-choice tests, variations on the traditional lecture format and evaluation of the student's progress. Simulations allow patients to experience the outcomes of health care decisions without putting themselves in danger. A simulation might, for example, allow diabetic patients to see what happens to their blood glucose when they change their medication, diet or exercise level.

Computer-based patient education is not yet in widespread use in primary care. Even in the United States a 1983 survey of 905 members of the American Academy of Family Physicians who used computers[4] found less than 4 per cent used them for patient education.

Nonetheless, there have been successful demonstrations of the value of computer-assisted instruction of patients. An early report from this field[4] investigated mid-stream urine specimens collected by young women after spoken, written, computer or no instructions. Computer instructions were found more effective than written instructions, and as good as or better than well-presented oral instructions in producing uncontaminated specimens. Computer-based lessons have been used to educate patients about the risk factors for ischaemic heart disease and to encourage behavioural change, and have been shown to result in increased knowledge. The Body Awareness Resource Network developed at the University of Wisconsin–Madison provides health information for adolescents. The Clinical Research Institute of Montreal has developed microcomputer-based educational question banks on a wide range of health and disease topics, and has obtained valuable feedback on the interests and concerns of patients seeking information from the banks. A number of computer applications have been developed for particular subjects, e.g. instructing patients about their renal failure,[6] lessons for sufferers from rheumatoid arthritis,[2] lessons to teach basic information about diabetes,[7] information about sexually transmitted disease,[8] dietary advice for patients with diabetes and limited educational background,[7] instructions for patients who need special diets.[5]

These examples give some flavour of the potential of computer-assisted learning. A number of the studies reported have shown enhancement of knowledge through computer-assisted learning. Those by Wheeler et al.[7] are particularly interesting in that they demonstrate that CAL may have clear advantages over traditional educational methods. There is a need for further rigorous comparison with established methods of teaching.

While CAL programs can be easily updated, one guideline for CAL instruction is that 100 hours of developer time are required to develop one hour of computer-based lesson material,[4] so certainly doctors who devise their own programs will find it a time-consuming if potentially rewarding task.

Nonetheless, there is a growing body of material available for use by patients and considerable future scope for CAL both in the education of patients about disease and in health education.

There is little doubt that CAL can 'dramatically improve the user's learning, retention, achievement and attitude',[9] and that it is 'an invaluable educational tool designed to make the health care professional's job easier and more effective'.[3]

Home computers

The applications discussed above have all been employed in a medical or paramedical environment, but we now live in a society where a great many individuals possess a personal microcomputer.

Software can be purchased off the shelf to educate both public and patients in their home environment. There are a considerable number of such programs available in the United States and some already in the United Kingdom, with wide variations in the quality of both the information and the instruction. Some of them facilitate home diagnosis, others give advice on diet and exercise, while other programs allow dietary analysis of food consumption.

Prestel

The British Telecom Prestel network is another source of publicly accessible health information in the United Kingdom. Meditel Ltd has responsibility for managing the information and delivering it through the network. Members of the public may subscribe to Prestel themselves, or make use of Prestel terminals operated by coin-in-the-slot mechanisms in public libraries. There are three choices of hardware for the private user: a dedicated Prestel terminal, a Prestel adaptor which will plug into a television set, or the addition of a modem to a microcomputer. In September 1986 there were some 65,000 terminals of all types attached to the network, about half of which were located in customers' homes.

While much of the medical information available through Prestel can only be accessed by health professionals, there is a substantial amount of information available to the general public, much of it supplied by the Health Education Council and the Department of Health and Social Security. Examples include information on health education, on vaccination, foreign travel and health, on health and safety, and services for the handicapped and social welfare. Various printed brochures on health issues can be ordered by use of response frames.

None of the frames on the Prestel medical data bases carries a frame charge, so the costs for private users consist of hardware costs, a quarterly subscription to Prestel, and telephone charges for calls to the nearest Prestel computer.

Some indication of how frequently these services are used is given by the figure of about 30,000 access counts in the medical field during August 1986, though many of these users would be health professionals rather than the lay public.

BROADCASTING

Teletext

A much more widely accessible potential source of health information in the United Kingdom is through the teletext services, the additional broadcast services of written and graphical information provided by the British Broadcasting Corporation and Independent Television. There are now some three million teletext television sets equipped with teletext decoders, which means that approximately nine to ten million people can receive the BBC's Ceefax or ITV's Oracle.[10,11] The number of households able to receive teletext transmissions is growing at a rate of over 70,000 a month, and it is predicted that by 1995 over 75 per cent of UK households will be equipped with teletext sets. Ceefax has some 600 pages of information available, while Oracle has around 1200 pages. Both contain magazine features and information services, so that for instance Ceefax has a consumer section which carries stories and tips on health, the items in which change each week. Typical examples might include a news story on the testing of a new pertussis vaccine, a guide on child safety in the home, and information about drug education packs aimed at 9–11-year-olds. In 1985–6 Ceefax provided 'a comprehensive guide to good health' (Fifteen Steps to Good Health) which was compiled in collaboration with the Health Education Council's Look After Yourself! project and broadcast over a 15-week period.

Closed-circuit broadcasting

The potential of communication via television and radio has also been realised in closed-circuit broadcasting within a hospital environment. Hyland[12] has reported on the use of radio by the dietitians of the Whittington Hospital to advise and educate hospital patients on aspects of human nutrition using London Hospitals Broadcasting, the third-largest commercial radio station in London. The message of the broadcasts was enhanced by distribution of booklets to the wards.

Extensive and developing use of health care information broadcasting in American hospitals has been described[13] with various national, regional and local networks supplying programmes to subscribing hospitals. Other institutions, rather than purchasing material from an outside source, produce all their own programmes. In addition to scheduled programming, some hospitals are also able to provide 'demand' programming, allowing patients to request particular videotapes when they wish. Increasingly, such facilities are seen as an integral part of a patient education programme, allowing patients to make better-informed decisions and undertake more responsibility for their own health.

Closed-circuit television and radio, of course, reach a relatively captive and possibly highly motivated audience. The more common situation, however, is that of mass communication to a potentially huge audience through public service broadcasting. Television in particular has immense potential power, having the essential characteristic that it is a visual medium so that it can preserve or transmit information as pictures and sound. The advantages it has over other media are that it can show movement and demonstrate human communicating behaviour. The juxtaposition of visual images and sound enables more information to be conveyed more quickly, and thus makes television and other visual media more powerful than radio.

PUBLIC SERVICE BROADCASTING

The health information available to patients described thus far has comprised that available either in a medical environment (hospitals and general practice) or through Prestel and teletext. For the majority of people, however, much of the information they receive about health and illness is provided by public service broadcasts either in the course of general programmes or through the broadcasting of special programmes concerned with health and illness.

Role of broadcasting

In 1976 the size of the audience for a BBC documentary broadcast at peak viewing time was estimated at five million,[14] with a three million audience for a documentary on BBC2. In 1978 it was stated that 'some five million people are likely to watch a medical programme'.[15] More recent viewing figures (1985–6) for medical programmes on both BBC and Independent Television range from 1.1 to 9.8 million with 'Medicine Now', a nationally broadcast radio programme, attracting an average audience of 0.6 million.

Furthermore, research suggests that the class profile of the audience for documentaries is usually similar to that of the whole population. The contribution of television and of public broadcasting as a whole is indeed potentially enormous because it can reach practically everyone.

This prospect of power elicits a variety of reactions from broadcasters, politicians and doctors.

In a random sample of 106 general practitioners in south-east Wales, 62 considered television the best method of informing the public about health care.[16] However, many doctors distrust journalists and producers,[16,17] because of past experience of sensational and simplistic treatment of medical stories, concentration on controversy, emphasis on curative and high-technology medicine, news items on the failures of medicine, and scare stores. An editorial in the *British Medical Journal* in 1975, recommending caution before doctors participate in television programmes, concludes 'it is "your words in their hands"'.[18] A famous subsequent cause for renewed distrust between the medical profession and the media was the controversial report on brain death shown on the current affairs programme 'Panorama'. Perhaps, therefore, some doctors would agree with the distinguished American television reporter Daniel Schorr: 'television lumbers into a complicated situation like King Kong, altering the landscape by its sheer weight and force'.[17]

But the case from the other side of the fence seems increasingly unanswerable. Maurice Macmillan MP,[19] writing 18 years ago of television as a generally accepted 'method of combining enjoyment with instruction', certainly felt that doctors were then lagging behind in making use of the broadcast media. 'They have tended to regard themselves rather more as witch doctors informing the ignorant savage than as leaders trying to bring a more educated and informed attitude to the people with whom they deal.' He pleaded for teachers who would bring understanding rather than experts laying down the law. In the same vein Fletcher,[20] writing as both doctor and broadcaster, says 'we have to discover techniques by which we can get our messages across without every viewer switching his set off or switching it over to another channel'.

There is, of course, great variety in both type of programme and message conveyed. The impact of fictional treatments of medicine should not be underrated. Early series such as 'Emergency Ward 10' and 'Dr Finlay's Casebook' are still remembered, and have spawned a number of successors with both hospital and community settings.

The main distinction in the subject-matter of non-fictional

programmes is between disease in its broadest sense and health, although there have also been programmes dealing with normal physiology. While David Cordingley, senior producer for health programmes in the BBC Continuing Education department, reckoned 'medicine had always been considered more sexy than health',[21] there has in this decade been a considerable change to a public health approach, in other words from information to exhortation, or 'from highbrow medicine to a "help yourself to health" approach'. It has been realised that there is 'more to medical/health programming than scientific research and political investigation'.

An important subgroup of broadcast programmes are those designed for use in schools.[22] Here too broadcasters have accepted their central public service role in health education, and for example of the 50 or so series on offer to schools from the IBA in 1987, eight are primarily designed as resources for health education.[23] The captive audience here is immense: one ITV programme, 'Good Health', was being used by 21 per cent of all primary and 15 per cent of all secondary schools in the UK in the spring term of 1986, and was thus reaching over a quarter of its available target audience of 8–12-year-olds.

Radio has the particular advantages over television of economy and of potentially very short lead-time in programme preparation. One remarkable use of local radio has been in contact tracing in collaboration with a local genito-urinary medicine clinic.[14]

A special additional category of broadcast programme is advertising, including public service advertising in the areas of health, safety and welfare produced by the Central Office of Information, and advertising produced by such bodies as the Health Education Council and the Scottish Health Education Unit.[22]

A comparatively recent development is the radio phone-in. An anecdotal account of a two-week London Broadcasting Company project in 1982 on 'Drugs and the family', in which seven hours of programming was backed up by 160 hours of 'off-air' counselling,[24] certainly suggests that there is a reservoir of need for such programmes from patients whose needs are not being met by their own doctors. The phone-in is for many a well-regarded and much-needed source of advice and information. Analysing the problems presented by callers on a regular medical open-line programme, Rogers[25] suggests 'local radio medical broadcasting may prove to be a useful preventive and educational tool as well as providing popular entertainment'.

Broadcasting support services

Increasingly, too, off-screen or off-the-air support is provided, so that the message of the programme or series can be reinforced. Indeed, the programme may become just one part of a multi-faceted health education campaign.

Barnes[26] has written of the ten-part BBC television series 'Play it Safe', broadcast in 1981, which dealt with the prevention of accidents to children. Planning for the programmes started almost two years beforehand, building on the existing close working relationships between the BBC Continuing Education Department and the Health Education Council and Scottish Health Education Group. 'The development of close co-operation was aided by the active willingness of the BBC Education staff to discuss with these agencies, well in advance, the priority areas of health care they had and to try to match these where appropriate by a broadcasting contribution'. Nonetheless, the producer still has to 'achieve a suitable balance between information, motivation and entertainment'.[26] In the 'Play it Safe' campaign, national television programmes, booklets and publicity materials were linked with a wide range of activities initiated and organised by local agencies throughout the country. The broadcasts were preceded ten months before transmission by 14 regional meetings to which local organisations and individuals with a role to play in the campaign were invited; and from six to four months before transmission by 40 local preview meetings at which the programmes were shown. Regular newsletters were distributed, 60,000 posters were sent out and 1½ million copies of a booklet, designed by the Health Education Council to support the series, were printed.

A similarly broad and more recent endeavour has been the BBC's 'Food and Health' campaign, launched in September 1985 with 'O'Donnell Investigates . . . Food and the Taste of Health', 'series showing that healthy eating can be affordable and fun'.[10] Books accompanying these series have sold over 170,000 copies, and 120,000 free health information packs were distributed in response to requests for programme follow-up material. The ensuing series, 'You Are What You Eat', attracted weekly audiences of up to 11 million, and 250,000 copies of the series booklet were sent out. Education officers of the BBC Educational Broadcasting Services department were much involved in preparation and support for the campaign, including the distribution of 50,000 posters.

The same public health approach, indeed one consciously

modelled on that of the BBC Continuing Education department, has been taken by Channel 4's commissioning editor for education.[21] Similarly, ITV Community Education Officers work to promote such programmes as ITV's 'Health and Family Matters' by contacting health professionals and others in advance of transmission, while back-up to Independent Local Radio broadcasts too 'can take the form of off-air telephone advice, information and referral services, and printed information to reinforce and expand on information given in the programme'.[23] Channel 4 has been particularly keen to back up programmes with leaflets and booklets.[27] One of their most popular pieces of print back-up has been on the 'Alexander Technique', when 11,388 copies were requested following a documentary which clearly excited considerable interest in an unfamiliar but highly effective approach to health. A 1986 IBA survey[23] found 10 per cent of the sample had sent for a free publication on health related to a television programme at least once. The BBC Research Department is currently investigating why people do or do not follow up broadcasts in this way, and how they change their behaviour as a result.

Of course, good intentions in developing support for broadcast programmes do not always succeed. One celebrated disaster was Granada's anti-smoking campaign on 'Reports Action', broadcast in October 1977, which offered viewers a free anti-smoking kit containing 'every known device to make you give it up and stop killing yourself', and said there was no need to rush as they had thousands. The item was 15 minutes long and drew what is said to have been the biggest response to a television programme in the history of broadcasting. 600,000 people asked for the kit, but Granada only had 10,000 available. Raw, who evaluated the programme, concluded 'this was grossly irresponsible broadcasting, which deliberately provoked a response for which there was totally inadequate backup'.[28]

Control of broadcasting

The British Broadcasting Corporation is governed by a Royal Charter which defines its objects, powers and obligations, its constitution and the sources and uses of its revenues. A Licence and Agreement, granted by the Home Secretary alongside the Charter, prescribes the terms and conditions of the Corporation's operations.[10]

Similarly, the Independent Broadcasting Authority fulfils the wishes of Parliament, as contained in the Broadcasting Act 1981, in providing television and radio services of information, education and entertainment additional to those of the BBC. It is the public body responsible for the organisation and supervision of the independent broadcasting system as a whole, and ensures that the services are of a high standard with a proper balance and wide range of subject-matter.[11]

Both the BBC and IBA necessarily have a system of review and reference to ensure impartiality and high standards, including the development of television programme guidelines and the scrutiny of advisory bodies. Article 9 of the Royal Charter allows the appointment of persons or committees to advise the Corporation, and since 1964 the BBC has had the benefit of advice from its Science Consultative Group, whose membership of twelve currently includes three doctors, one of whom is a general practitioner.[10] Similarly, the Medical Advisory Panel of the IBA, which scrutinises advertisements for medicines and treatments, contains eleven consultants, including eight doctors of whom one is a family doctor.[11]

The IBA's Television Programme Guidelines state:

> for programmes on medical subjects it is necessary to obtain competent professional advice; and on matters of potential controversy to give a hearing to more than one opinion. There are some subjects, such as cancer or certain aspects of mental health, that are particularly sensitive. A soundly-based unsensational but informative programme can do a genuine service. But in order to avoid unnecessary distress it is essential to handle with care any information about controversial or novel forms of treatment, or criticisms, explicit or implicit, of current medical practice. Equal care must be exercised in fictional programmes in which medical matters are featured.

Expert medical guidance is similarly sought by the BBC, not only for documentaries and current affairs programmes but for drama programmes such as 'East Enders'. The *IBA Guidelines* and Independent Local Radio Programming Notes of Guidance also deal amongst other matters with smoking and drinking, drug-taking and solvent abuse, the wearing of seatbelts and tobacco sponsorship.

Nevertheless within this overall advisory structure the actual selection and production of programmes places a considerable amount of power in the hands of individual producers and presenters. A television editor writes that 'the way programmes are chosen may on the surface seem almost random. The system really relies on individual producers and individual programme editors remaining sufficiently in touch and using their judgement. Basically a producer and editor can only follow his own nose.'[14]

MASS COMMUNICATION CAMPAIGNS

In contrast to the information conveyed in individual programmes on radio and television, to which members of the public can decide themselves whether to tune in or not, health campaigns involving mass communication aim to saturate a population with health and illness information in an attempt to induce a change of behaviour.

Tones[23] has described five stages which are necessary before a health promotion programme can succeed; namely increasing awareness, promoting understanding, increasing motivation, acquisition of skills, and continuing support.

He argues that it is difficult for mass media to promote understanding of complex information, and to persuade people to change their attitude and behaviour unless they are already favourably disposed to the change. Nor can mass media easily offer the support needed by individuals who have made often difficult lifestyle changes. On the other hand mass media have an important 'agenda-setting' role. They may not be especially good at telling people what to think, but they are extraordinarily successful in telling people what to think about.

It is becoming increasingly clear that success in achieving behavioural change is unlikely to occur with a mass media campaign alone. It requires a properly integrated programme having a sound education infrastructure[23] and preferably additional community support.[29]

In spite of these difficulties some outstandingly successful campaigns have been reported. In the Stanford Heart Disease Prevention Project[16,30] a 25–30 per cent reduction in coronary heart disease risk was achieved in the sample population compared with a 2 per cent risk reduction in the control population. Following the North Karelia Project in Finland,[23,31] which included social engineering strategies and involvement of a wide range of agencies in a community effort, there was a decrease in coronary mortality of 24 per cent in men and 51 per cent in women between 1969 and 1979 in North Karelia compared with a 12 per cent and 24 per cent decline in Finland as a whole. A number of current initiatives have built on the experience gained in these projects, including the Welsh Heart Programme.[23]

CONCLUSION

Broadcasting and the more recent availability of computers provide immense opportunities for increasing knowledge and influencing attitudes. The widespread availability of home computers, video-cassette recorders and the future introduction of cable and satellite television provide further opportunities to reach small audiences at low cost, which have not yet been realised.

Nonetheless, while computers as a medium for health education have largely remained under the control of doctors, most patients can learn more about health and prevention of illness through the printed word and particularly through the broadcast media.

Doctors should regard these media as allies rather than threats, should co-operate and become involved with radio and television so that the information and advice presented are accurate, informed and appropriate. This plea was made some years ago when the medical profession was more conservative and even actively hostile to the notion of lay journalists having control of medical messages,[19,20] but it is equally timely today.

Finally there is urgent need for an extension of studies into the economics and effectiveness of the use of the media in health education. It seems clear that, while the mass media can set the agenda and increase the level of awareness, behavioural change is more likely to occur when mass communication exercises are reinforced by a community-based approach and communication at an individual level.

REFERENCES

1. Dove, G. (1978) The psychotropic computer. *World Medicine*. 6 September, pp. 81–5
2. Wetstone, S.L., Sheehan, T.J., Votaw, R.G., Peterson, M.G. and Rothfield, N. (1985) Evaluation of a computer based education lesson for patients with rheumatoid arthritis. *Journal of Rheumatology*, *12*, 907–12
3. Cohen, J. (1985) Computers in patient education. *Computer*, *77*, 71–2

4. Ellis, L.B.M. (1985) Computer-based patient education. *Primary Care*, *12*, 547–55

5. Williams, C.S. and Burnet, L.W. (1984) Future applications of the micro-computer in dietetics. *Human Nutrition: Applied Nutrition*, *38A*, 99–109

6. Bryant, Y. (1985) Soft cells. *Nursing Times*, 24 April, p. 18

7. Wheeler, L.A., Wheeler, M.L., Ours, P. and Swider, C. (1985) Evaluation of computer-based diet education in persons with diabetes mellitus and limited educational background. *Diabetes Care*, *8*, 537–44

8. Deardoff, W.W. (1986) Computerized health education: a comparison with traditional formats. *Health Education Quarterly*, *13*, 61–72

9. Williams, P.H. and Loder, N.C. (1984) Microcomputer: educational tool for clinical practitioners and clients. *Medical Informatics (London)*, *9*, 314–15

10. *BBC Annual Report and Handbook 1987* (1986) British Broadcasting Corporation, London

11. Melaniphy, M. (ed.) (1987) *Television and radio*. Independent Broadcasting Authority, London

12. Hyland, K.M. (1980) Nutrition broadcasting. *Journal of Human Nutrition*, *34*, 52–3

13. Brown, M.S. (1984) A review of health care television programming. *Hospitals*, 16 December, pp. 88–9

14. Goodchild, P. (1976) The role and responsibility of the mass media in the UK. In: Catterall, R.D. and Nicol, C.S. (eds), *Sexually transmitted diseases*. Academic Press, London, pp. 245–50

15. Swann, Sir M. (1978) Television medicine. *British Medical Journal*, *1*, 1274–5

16. Smail, S.A. (1985) Medicine and the media. *Journal of the Royal College of General Practitioners*, *35*, 363–4

17. Bedford, R. (1979) Medicine and the media: the need to strengthen the bridge. *Journal of the Royal College of Physicians of London*, *13*, 7–10, 14

18. Medicine on television (1975) *British Medical Journal*, *1*, 539

19. Macmillan, M. (1969) The future of television and medicine. *Proceedings of the Royal Society of Medicine*, *62*, 401–2

20. Fletcher, C.M. (1969) Health education. *Proceedings of the Royal Society of Medicine*, *62*, 398–9

21. Harbord, J. (1985) A taste of our own medicine . . . Broadcast, 6 September

22. Thomson of Monifieth, Lord (1981) Health education and the media. *Independent Broadcasting*, *29*, 13–16

23. Various authors (1987) *Health Trends*. *19*, 16–19, 20–2, 23–7, 28–30

24. Webb, P. (1983) Hooked on radio. *Journal of the Royal Society of Health*, *103*, 174–80

25. Rogers, A. (1980) Doctor on the air. *Journal of the Royal College of General Practitioners*, *30*, 629–31

26. Barnes, N. Play it safe. *Media in Education and Development*, *3*, 43–5

27. Smail, S.A. (1983) Doctor on the air. *The Practitioner, 227,* 1839–45

28. Karpf, A. (1981) A case of, don't do as I do. Broadcast, 20 April.

29. Katz, D. (1985) Cable television and health promotion: a feasibility study with arthritis patients. *Health Education Quarterly, 12,* 379–89

30. Alcalay, R. (1983) The impact of mass communication campaigns in the health field. *Social Science and Medicine, 17,* 87–94

31. Williams, B.T. (1984) Are public health education campaigns worth while? *British Medical Journal, 288,* 170–1

Part 4

In the Pipeline

10

Clinical Information and Data Bases

Ellie Scrivens and Claudine Hornyold-Strickland

Before we describe how the development of data bases may affect general practitioners in their work, which is the purpose of this chapter, it will be helpful to review the present position.

DEFINITIONS AND FORMATS

A single collection of information in computerised form is usually called a data base.[1] All data bases consist of two components: the first is the hardware on which the information is stored, together with the method by which the information is accessed; the second is the nature of the information which is stored, the content of the data base. With regard to medical data bases the physical component ranges from a floppy disc used on a microcomputer in a surgery or hospital to the large hard disc memory of a distant mainframe computer accessed through telephone lines, cable or satellite. The content may relate to any aspect of medical practice. In general practice, for example, the information might be that collected 'in-house' such as patients' medical records, or provided by external agencies such as information about medical procedures, therapeutics or diseases.

Data bases are available in different formats: on-line, videotex, floppy disc (magnetic medium for micros, used for storing and transferring software and data), CD-ROMS (compact disc–read only memory). These formats form a continuum of service, and therefore usefulness, for the user. Floppy discs are very limited in the amount of information to which the user has access. The data base is limited to that which can be stored on a disc at the time of purchase; although more information can be added by the purchaser this is not necessarily easy.

CD-ROMS store large volumes of information but are essentially fixed in format and content and cannot therefore be updated or enlarged.

A more attractive format is videotex. In its limited form this is a system that uses a combination of existing telephone (for connection to a data base) and television (for display). These technologies provide low-cost access to large volumes of remotely stored information. The main example of this in the UK is Prestel. To maintain low costs, access is slow and restricted in function. An elaboration of the system allows 'closed user groups' where some subscribers have access to information not generally available to others. The data base provides a general information service: for example, Glaxo provides a drug information service.

Videotex can be adapted to provide interactive facilities. It can be used to store, update and communicate information. For example, a number of Health Authorities use the system to store and communicate limited information of local use within their own districts. However, access to these systems tend to be inefficient and expensive if the volume of two-way, interactive communication is large.

The most useful format is one which allows complete interaction between the user and the data base. That is, the user can direct the way in which the data are accessed and under appropriate conditions can add to or modify the contents of the data base. In general the user requires a terminal which is connected to the host computer on which the data base is stored, most commonly using the telephone system. The cost of access to data bases varies according to the host's computer, but it is mainly a function of the time connection and (because of the charging structure of telephone companies) distance from the host computer. In order to keep the level of costs incurred in accessing data bases down, 'gateway' services can be used. These provide the user with connection to one or more host computers, for the same level of cost as if all were local.

THE NATURE OF THE INFORMATION STORED

Information stored in data bases consists of three major types: reference data, source data and local data.

Reference data bases

These data bases store references to medical publications. The data bases contain citations, abstracts, journal information, dissertations and conference proceedings. The purpose is to enable rapid and easy access to the location of medical knowledge — an electronic version of the familiar methods of cataloguing published information as used in libraries. The computerised reference data base has advantages over its manual counterpart. It can be readily and easily updated, keeping up with the pace of developments in any field. Examples of such data bases are Medline, the electronic version of *Index Medicus*, and Embase, the version of *Excerpta Medica*. Electronic systems are in some instances now replacing paper systems. For example, the *Medical Research Directory*, a compilation of research in UK universities, hospitals and government establishments, is only accessible electronically.

Source data bases

These data bases can store the full text of journal articles, textbooks and conference proceedings, etc., or compilations of information such as directories or compendia. Unlike the reference data base which simply indicates the existence and the location of information as a library catalogue, the source data base holds detailed information, such as the content of published papers, the electronic equivalent of a journal or reference book or compilations of information. Well-used examples are Martindale On-line which provides evaluated information on drugs (extra pharmacopoeia) and RTCES, the Registry of Drug Data Bases.

A number of companies have been set up to collect and store information which is of interest to professional groups. For example one company, Meditel, provides an information service for those working in medicine. Meditel collects and organises a wide range of information of interest to the medical profession. The information is constantly updated and subscribers have access to the stores of information. A number of companies provide data bases holding current information about developments in, for example, professional practice, and research which can be accessed through videotex and on-line facilities.

Drug data bases

Drug data bases are the type of source data base most frequently used by the profession at present. They fall into three principal categories:

1. Drug evaluations: these provide evaluation information on such things as adverse reactions, contraindications and drug interactions for selected drugs on the market.
2. Drug therapy: these provide comparisons and evaluation information on selected classes of drugs.
3. Drug abuse: these provide general information on treatment and on practices concerning drug and alcohol abuse.

A number of drug data bases are now available to GPs through a number of systems which are listed in Table 10.1.

Access to large-scale data bases allows GPs to gain useful information on drugs. However, the benefit is not all one-way. In a number of cases pharmaceutical companies have been able to take advantage of the interactive nature of their data bases to monitor the effects of their drugs. For example, in the USA some GPs are connected to the computer host of major pharmaceutical companies and through a videotex terminal input data from patients who are taking the drug. A large-scale study of one drug being taken by 25,000 patients is being conducted by the pharmaceutical company Squibb.

Similar research is being conducted in the UK.

Local data bases

The third type of data base which is of importance in general practice is the bank of data obtained from local information; for example, patients' records, Health Authority and hospital activity information, local social services information. The data in these data bases obviously cannot be purchased but are compiled from information collected from within the practice and from local sources.

The compilation of a practice register data base has been the foundation of general practice computing in the UK. To the basic details of all patients registered with the practice other items are usually added to enable the data base to be used for a variety of programmes. Four of the larger software companies have developed programs which allow analyses of epidemiological trends within the

Table 10.1: Drug data bases available to GPs

(a) On-line systems

Name	Information producers	Availability
AMA/Net drug evaluation	American Medical Association, USA	GTE telenet, Medical Information Network, Easy Net
AMA/Net drug therapy	American Medical Association, USA	GTE telenet, Medical Information Network, Easy Net
Deltabank	Databank: St Luke Hospital, Surrey	Data Star Easy Net
Drug Info/ Alcohol Use and Abuse	Drug Information Service Center, Minneapolis, USA	BRS, BRS/BRKTHRU
Drug Information full text	American Society of Hospital Pharmacists	BRS BRS/BRKTHRU
International Pharmaceutical	American Society of Hospital Pharmacists	BLAISELINK, BRS BRS/after dark BRS/BRKTHRU Dialog, Easy Net, ESA-IRS
Martindale On-line	Pharmaceutical Society of Great Britain	Data Star, Easy Net
Mental Health Abstracts	IFI/Plenum Data Company USA	BRS BRS/BRKTHRU (1969–81) Data Star (1969–80) Dialog, Easy Net
Merck Index	Merck and Company	BRS, BRS/Saunders Colleague, Telesystemes-Questel
Pharmaprojects	Pharmaprojects, Richmond, Surrey	Data-Star Easy Net
Pharmline	National Health Service, Regional Information	Data-Star Easy Net
RTECS Registry of Toxic Effects of Chemical Substances	National Institute for Occupational Safety and Health	BLAISELINK Chemical information system DIMDI

(b) Videotex data bases

Name	Availability
Doctel/MSD Foundation	Prestel/Datel CUG p35066600
Glaxo Laboratories Drug Therapy	Prestel/BMJ GLAXO CUG p265
ICI Pharmaceutical ICI Division	Prestel/ICI CUG p42499
May and Baker	Prestel/Viewtel p2028411
Medicine in the News	Prestel/Meditel CUG p567470
Stuart Pharmaceutical Ltd	Prestel/Meditel CUG p56721

practice population. Further description as to the way these local data bases are commonly used can be found in Chapter 8.

FUTURE DEVELOPMENTS

Given the pace of technological change, it seems certain that in five to ten years time the working environment of a GP will be very different from today. The pressures for change in other areas are described elsewhere in this section. The developments which can be expected with respect to clinically related data bases will be described for each type of data base in turn.

Reference data bases

These will undoubtedly become more available, with faster access and greater selectivity geared towards specific client groups. The technology already exists, but until now general practitioners have been a very small and commercially unimportant group. As the number of computerised practices increases worldwide this picture will change.

Source data bases

This is the area where the greatest changes can be expected to occur. In the field of clinical medicine source data bases have taken a long time to appear. Until recently such data bases were only produced in the USA, almost entirely by researchers for their own use. These data bases have largely proved inappropriate for easy use by GPs. Researchers tend to work in a specific field, often over a long period of time, and to structure their information in a similar way. In contrast GPs require quick and easy access to a data base which contains information on a wide range of subjects. Today this situation is changing and some data base constructors are now designing source data bases tailor-made for use by general practitioners.

One British example is the Oxford System of Medicine (OSM), which is being produced by the Oxford University Press in co-operation with the Imperial Cancer Research Fund Biomedical Computing Unit.[2] This project aims to provide general practitioners with very fast access to the equivalent of a large medical library. In addition it is planned to include the facility for providing prompts, listing decision options and providing the equivalent of a second opinion. More radical developments are also occurring which could allow access to vast amounts of data collected by GPs, and which reflect not the structured and restricted work of researchers but, more importantly, the reality and the necessary pragmatism of the work of the GP. In a pilot study started in February 1987 Vamp is collecting and amalgamating data from GP computer users which have been generated in the course of their normal daily work. Analysis of such data and their subsequent availability with a clinical data base has enormous potential.

In the field of therapeutics also source data bases based on GP experience are being developed.

Local data bases

It can also be confidently predicted that the amount and scope of information available in practice data bases, both that generated within the practice and from local professional sources, will transform the patient record and the information available through use of the record within the forseeable future.[3] This aspect is discussed more fully in Chapter 12.

CONCLUSIONS

In the past GPs have suffered from limited access to published information only being able to find information through journals, libraries or empirical research. In the near future it seems probable that they will be swamped by ever-increasing sources of information. One of the most highly prized skills of the future will be selecting the most appropriate source of data to meet particular needs. GPs will be offered a wide range of data bases to choose from, for access to which they will be charged. Making the wrong choice may therefore prove an expensive mistake. The cost of using the data bases, and the quality of the information it offers, will become as common a practice management problem as is the decision about which microcomputer to buy today.

Ready access to large-scale data bases could revolutionise the way in which GPs work, though like all professionals affected by the information revolution, GPs will need to have a very clear picture of their information needs and of the effects information will have on their professional practices.

REFERENCES

1. Cowie, A. and Duckitt, P. (1986) *Computer based sources of information in Medicine*. Royal College of Physicians, London
2. Oxford System of Medicine (1986) *Demonstration of an experimental prototype*. Oxford University Press, Oxford
3. White, D.H. (1984) The computer health check — the first 100 patients. *Journal of the Royal College of General Practitioners*, *34*, 661-3

11

Aids to Diagnosis — an Impertinent Look at Some Pertinent Questions

Tim de Dombal

INTRODUCTION

The chosen title for this presentation — an impertinent look at some pertinent questions — may well be facile, but it is far from being flippant. For it encapsulates two important concepts which have combined to hold back the development of computing in general practice for many years.

First, the word 'impertinent' reflects a total non-meeting of minds between doctors and computer people dating back to the 1960s — and to some extent the fault of both 'sides'. 'Impertinent' computer people appeared in the 1960s — waving printout around like some papal encyclical and declaring that it was time for medicine to be 'rationalised' (whatever that meant). Their missionary zeal in promoting their own technology was only matched (and indeed exceeded) by the zeal with which doctors defended their interests. Superficially, the medical profession were successful — in that the perceived challenge of the computer and its high priests were both driven off — but this Pyrrhic victory proved to be to the eventual benefit of neither the doctor, nor the patient, nor the public purse.

The word 'pertinent' is also selected with some care. For this reflects another major failing which has proved of considerable detriment over the years — namely a failure of both groups of combatants to inform themselves about the *pertinent* questions which concern the introduction of computers into clinical practice. To some extent it is easier in hindsight to look kindly upon the doctors in this respect. Computer people tended to ignore medical ways because they wanted to change them. Doctors ignored the computer simply because they knew next to nothing about it.

Times have changed. Whereas in the 1950s and 1960s (when

many clinical practitioners qualified in clinical medicine) the computer was almost non-existent. Nowadays between 10 and 20 per cent of doctors' homes have (a) some kind of personal computer system and (b) at least one offspring quite capable of running it (to whom computer illiteracy is almost as difficult to understand as the inability to drive a car).

In seeking reasons for this technological change, and for the rapid introduction of computers into clinical medicine, it is customary to speak of the rapid development of microcomputer technology and of relatively sudden financial stringencies which have overtaken clinical practice in all its forms. Actually, however, neither of these two reasons fully explains the situation or explains why computer-aided decision support has become not simply a rather good idea but *fundamentally necessary* to the practice of good clinical medicine.

The reason why computers have now such an important role to play in medicine is exactly the same as the reason why they have become indispensable in areas of life such as banking and airline travel. For in many walks of life — including clinical medicine — the field has become so complex, the amount of information needed to operate effectively within it so large, as to render totally and utterly inappropriate current and more traditional ways of storing and retrieving information. Indeed, what information science contributes to the problem — more than anything else — is that the problem of 'keeping up with current medicine' is of such magnitude that the introduction of computers is *necessary* and *inevitable* rather than desirable.

This may sound like yet another diatribe against the poor clinician — another plea for his or her replacement by automated systems, another attack upon personalised clinical care. It is nothing of the sort. Computers will never in our working lifetime *replace* the caring, concerned clinicians — and neither should they do so. But just as the general practitioner has harnessed other developments of a technological nature to assist in daily work, so must the computer be harnessed to the GPs plough — to assist rather than replace or threaten. This should not prove impossible. Most GPs have managed to harness a whole series of technological innovations to assist them in their work — from the telephone through the ECG to the motor car — yet few nowadays feel threatened by them.

The problem is, however, that whilst most sensible doctors are only too happy to harness whatever technology they can get their hands on to help with the formidably difficult task of clinical decision-making and diagnosis, many are quite unable so to harness computers, since the doctors lack basic information which may enable them to make up their minds as to the value of the technology. In short, they don't know the answers to some pertinent questions — what do we mean by diagnosis?, what do we mean by automated diagnostic processes or information technology?, do we need it on *a priori* grounds?, what is available and does it work?, what are the problems and counter-arguments?

The purpose of the remaining paragraphs in this chapter is to set out these pertinent questions and attempt answers for at least some of them.

WHAT DO WE MEAN BY DIAGNOSIS?

Medical diagnosis has been variously described over the years as an art, a skill, a science and a technique. In recent years a whole industry (often referred to as process tracing) has grown up centred on the problem of what doctors actually do when they make a diagnosis. The results of this process have turned out to be predictable, but important in what is to follow — and it is therefore worth spending some time upon the question, just what do we mean by 'diagnosis'?

The first point to emerge from studies in the 1960s was that whatever diagnosis was it was *not* simply a matter of tying labels on patients. (Most GPs are aware of this, but the point is important since most computer people weren't.) Hence the systems of the 1960s were designed to 'do diagnosis' and take over the doctor's role — as if that were all there was to clinical medicine and its practice!

Gradually, over a period of about ten years, workers in the field ceased to talk of 'diagnosis' and began to speak of 'the diagnostic process' a three-part activity which involves:

(a) obtaining information from patients;
(b) analysing it in the hope of identifying the cause of the problem; and
(c) finally deciding what to do about it.

(These points are reflected in Figure 11.1).

Next, it became quite clear that 'diagnosis' — like happiness in the song — means different things to different people. How convenient it would be for computer people if we all did things the same

Figure 11.1: The diagnostic process

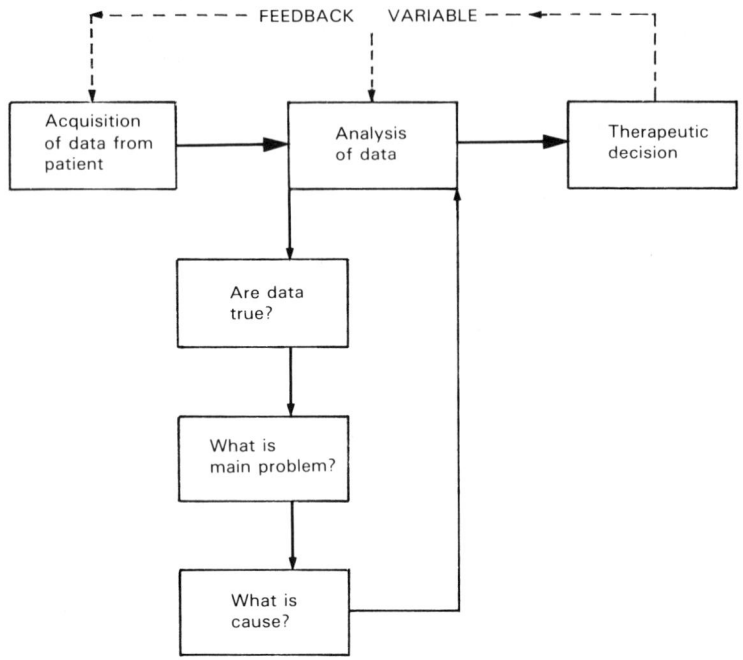

way each time. Of course, this is not the case; doctors differ from each other in the way they approach a problem. Two doctors will approach the same case in quite different ways. Worse, the same doctor will approach different cases in different ways, and it has simply proved quite impossible to 'model' the diagnostic process as a monolithic structure which all doctors will follow, other than in the very broad terms of Figure 11.1.

So, for the purposes of the present discussion, there is

unfortunately no such thing as a great universal diagnostic process, which we all follow (or more sinisterly which we can all be *made* to follow). All one can say about 'diagnosis' is that most doctors collect information from patients, analyse it and decide what to do, but outside these terms each doctor will work out his or her own salvation each time round, modifying technique as a result of increasing experience, so that the procedure adopted in a given patient is that most appropriate to the case.

DO WE NEED HELP?

Of course it can be argued cogently that, although clinical practice is becoming more complex, (and the amount of medical knowledge potentially available to the doctor expanding in exponential fashion), this does not affect the individual doctor. Complexity is an interesting facet of life, but not one which affects day-to-day medical care.

Unfortunately, such a cosy concept does not fit in with observed fact. Results of studies conducted in the past 20 years or so have revealed absolutely no grounds for complacency on this issue. These studies indicate that the net effect of the complex problems discussed has proved to be little short of catastrophic in day-to-day clinical care. Studies have indicated what appears to be a dramatic decline in the quality of what might be termed 'traditional' areas of clinical interview and examination — and it is difficult to avoid the conclusion that with the 'high-tech' brand of medicine now practised, many doctors have lost or forgotten at least some of their traditional clinical skills.

Thus studies have clearly shown that doctors nowadays do not elicit data at all well from patients. They tend to ask large numbers of questions which are not relevant to a given situation[1] — often at the expense of questions which *are* relevant to that situation.[2] In one study, no less than one question in five put by the doctor to the patient was so vaguely phrased that three other doctors observing the interview independently could not agree which question had been asked; whilst one in six patient responses was so vague that the same three observers could not agree whether the patient had said 'yes' or 'no'.[3]

Not surprisingly, doctors tend to get confused as a result! They ignore clues to diagnosis which are, with the advantage of hindsight, obvious;[4] sometimes because they overlook them, but often

Table 11.1: Results of initial investigations made regarding a 31-year-old woman with chronic abdominal pain

Haemoglobin: 9.7 g/dl
Erythrocyte sedimentation rate: 2 mm/h
Blood film examination: mild stippling
Reticulocyte count: 3 per cent
White cell count: 6.5×10^9/l, with normal differential
Platelets: 360×10^9/l
Clotting screen: normal

Plasma sodium: 135 mmol/l
Plasma potassium: 3.4 mmol/l
Urea: 7.1 mmol/l
Random blood sugar: 4.5 mmol/l
Liver function tests: normal
Creatinine: 103 μmol/l
Creatinine clearance: 48 ml/min
Urinary protein: 0.13 g/24 h
Albumin: 44 g/l
Calcium: 2.3 mmol/l
Phosphate: 0.97 mmol/l
Autoantibody screen (including acetylcholine receptor antibodies): negative
Protein electrophoresis and immunoglobulins: normal
Thyroxine: 115 nmol/l
Serum copper: 18.4 μmol/l
Caeruloplasmin: 2.5 μmol/l
Serum iron: 25 μmol/l
Total iron-binding capacity: 55 μmol/l
Serum zinc: 15 μmol/l
Serum vitamin B12: 400 μg/ml
Red cell folate: 578 ng/ml
Phytanic acid: negative
Urine arsenic: not detected
Microscopy of urine: no cells revealed
Urinary glycine excretion: elevated
Urinary porphyrin screen: slightly increased urobilinogen, positive for uroporphyrin and coproporphyrin
Porphobilinogen: negative
TRH test: flattened TSH response with max. 4.4 mU/l at 60 min
FSH/HRH stimulation: normal response

X-rays (chest, abdomen, knees and elbows): normal
Intravenous pyelogram: normal
Electromyography: normal motor and sensor conduction; repetitive stimulation: normal
Electroencephalogram: normal
CT scan of head with view of pituitary fossa: normal

because doctors simply do not know what clues to look for.[5] Finally, and particularly overseas, doctors obtain relatively large quantities of relatively useless biochemical data (see Table 11.1 for a prime example of this tendency), and when they get it they utilise less than 5 per cent of the biochemical data they have requested.[6]

Again, it should be stressed that this set of considerations is of intense practical consequence. Studies of performance have shown, again and again, that these problems lead to poor decision-making. As regards acute abdominal pain, studies have repeatedly shown that the diagnostic accuracy in hospital at first clinical contact is less than 50 per cent.[7] In many studies perforation rates for appendicitis exceed 25 per cent (and it has recently been shown that perforation of an appendix in a young woman increases four-fold the chance of tubal infertility),[8] whilst in many centres, negative laparotomy rates exceed 50 per cent. Nor is the problem confined to hospital. MacAdam[5] showed in a remarkable study that the 'lead time' between presentation to the GP with symptoms due to gastrointestinal cancer and establishment of the diagnosis varied between 24 weeks and 46 weeks according to the area of the gastrointestinal tract involved by the cancer.

Any argument, therefore, which suggests that the current problems which arise in handling data in modern clinical practice are immaterial rests on very shaky foundations indeed. One may argue about ways of rectifying the problem — but all the available evidence suggests that current problems in assimilating information have a profound and harmful effect upon performance at the clinical level, both inside and outside hospital.

CAN INFORMATION SCIENCE ASSIST US?

It is, however, a considerable step from admitting that we need help (which seems to be the case) and asserting that the computer has come, or will come, to our salvation (which is a claim often made by computer buffs, but for which there is relatively little evidence to date). In particular, it is necessary to distinguish between computer technology and information science, and to look at the different areas of the diagnostic process separately.

Information collection

Considering the 'grand design' of the diagnostic process (Figure 11.1) it seems reasonable to look in turn at each of the main areas of this process. Thus considering first the problem of data collection, computer systems have already been designed to achieve this in an automated fashion. Perhaps the most notable of these systems is the Glasgow Dyspepsia system (GLADYS).[9] This system carries out a detailed interview with patients suffering from dyspepsia, and subsequently compares the resulting interview data with a data base of information about several hundred other cases.

This system is perhaps of special interest because of early studies carried out in which the patients' reactions to such a system were assessed. These proved to be illuminating — not least because the patients' perception of the computer system was in many cases that it had insight into their problem, was sympathetic to them — and in many cases was compared favourably on each of these scores with the doctor who eventually saw the patient, a swingeing indictment of current medical practice if ever there was one.

Clearly, therefore, computer systems *can* be designed which can elicit data from patients with more or less the same effectiveness as a doctor. However, it needs to be stressed that the Glasgow system operated in an area of clinical medicine where the interview with the patient is of paramount importance — and in other areas of medicine one might expect the computer to be less effective. (It is not difficult to foresee grave problems, for example, in attempting such an interview with a patient suffering from acute pain — and even more problem in attempting to replace the traditional forms of physical examination.) Moreover, it is clear that an experienced doctor will obtain much information from a patient by a 'gestalt' process, by subconsciously reacting to the patient's 'manner' — particularly if the patient is already known to the doctor — in a way that no computer program currently constructed can mimic.

It thus seems that computer technology can be of some help in data collection — but this help is restricted to specific areas of clinical practice. Nonetheless, the difficulties outlined above do point to a major role for *information science* in data collection. Information science (as opposed to computer technology) studies the way information is transmitted and received; and in this instance it would appear that there is great scope for clarification of terminology and for deciding just what questions *are* vital to a particular area of clinical practice. This is moreover an area where practising clinicians have an important role to play; a point which will be discussed in more detail later on.

Analysis of patient information

Turning to the *analysis* of the information which the doctor receives from the patient, Figure 11.1 indicates that there are three essential steps to this process. First, the doctor needs to decide whether the patient is telling the 'truth' or not. Quite apart from the obvious problems of malingering, the doctor needs to decide what the patient's problem actually is. (For example, a patient may complain of fatigue and weight loss — and only on supplementary questioning will a recent alternation in bowel habit be elicited, giving the essential clue to the diagnosis of colorectal cancer.)

Deciding whether the patient is telling the truth, and deciding what the patient's problem really is, are relatively well done by most doctors at the present time. Of more importance, they are both surprisingly *badly* done by present-day computer systems. Quite apart from the obvious problems (as Arthur C. Clarke sagely remarks, it is easy to design a computer system which is *fool*-proof, but very difficult to design one which is proof against *malice*), computers are spectacularly bad at 'latching on to' significant clues of low probability. (Certainly, ferreting out the 'true problem' which lies behind what the patient is actually saying is currently quite beyond computer systems.)

The corollary of this is that at present one can do no more than suggest a relatively restricted role for the computer. Instead of trying to take on the mantle of a surrogate doctor, all computers can do at present is to adopt a much more subjunctive role. That is to say, once the doctor has obtained information from the patient, *and* has decided that the information is 'true' *and* has decided in broad outline what the patient's problem is — then the computer may be called into play. The computer may then (once this initial groundwork has been achieved) be used to discriminate between some common causes of the patient's particular problem — by comparing the patient's symptoms with those of a large series of other patients with the same problem — and suggest a possible diagnosis, or series of diagnoses, to the doctor.

Such a system might well be very useful and welcome to the doctor concerned. But it in no way represents 'doing diagnosis' — nor should it be so represented. All that is being achieved is to fit the computer in to an existing diagnostic process — just as one would fit in an ECG analysis or a blood test. Indeed, many sensible computer people and doctors now view the computer in this restricted light. Just as one would analyse the patient's white blood cells by turning to an automated system, or the patient's heart electrical impulses by turning to an ECG machine, one turns to the computer for similar predictive information — to be weighed against the rest of the evidence by the only person capable of looking at the whole picture, the doctor in charge of the case.

Decision-making

Making decisions is a topic considered elsewhere in this volume — but since it is an integral part of the diagnostic process, and since one cannot entirely separate diagnosis and decision-making, some brief remarks may be appropriate here.

Many doctors would argue that unless a totally unforeseen breakthrough occurs within our working lifetime, clinical decisions should be the responsibility of clinicians and not computers. This is not simply Luddism — there is much to support this point of view. Perhaps the biggest problem of all hangs over the question of 'utility' of treatment.

Whatever the doctor does, and whatever the outcome, that outcome will have a certain 'utility' to the patient (and the patient to society). But the most formidable difficulties remain over assigning weightings, or numerical values, to these outcomes. Consider, for example, the 'value' of a negative laparotomy. To a young healthy adult male the 'negative benefit' (the term often employed) of a negative laparotomy may be minimal. The risk is not great, the scar no great handicap — it is even possible to win an Olympic marathon three weeks later (Tokyo, 1960). Yet to a young girl bothered about her appearance, or a haemophiliac, or an old person with COAD, the 'harm' done by this unnecessary operation is much greater. But exactly how much? What mathematical value should we assign to this harm, and how should we go about adding it up? Whose opinion should we take? (The doctor's or the patient's attitudes may differ radically, and often do.[10])

Until such questions are answered, information technology, many would argue, can only wait in the wings; and it may be a very long time before computer-based systems begin to make decisions about patients.

The upshot of all of this is to suggest once again a fairly restricted role for computer-aided diagnostic systems. Possibly of value in some areas of medicine in helping to secure information from patients, their principal use in the foreseeable future would seem to be in a role analogous to other special investigations, that is to say in helping the doctor by providing additional assistance once the doctor has already collected information, has decided that it represents the 'truth', and has decided on the patient's main problem. The computer can then analyse the information, and suggest some possible diagnoses to the doctor, so that the doctor in turn can make a better-informed decision about treatment.

This is a far cry from the computer systems of fiction; and it is a far cry from the 'big brother'-type systems which aim to replace the doctor as both diagnostician and decision-maker, and of which many doctors are (understandably) apprehensive. It is, however, a role for the computer which is perhaps both more practical and more acceptable — and in the ensuing section we shall assess whether in this more restricted role the computer has any role to play.

DOES INFORMATION SCIENCE ASSIST US?

If we are talking in terms of computer systems which mimic doctors — and deal with the whole of medicine — then for reasons already outlined, the answer must be 'no'. In the past decade or so, however, computer systems have begun to emerge which offer some hope that we can expect to derive some help from small, simple systems designed to aid the doctor in the management of specific areas of clinical medicine.

Perhaps the best example of such a system is the computer-aided diagnostic system first devised in Leeds, and later tested round the world, designed to aid doctors in the diagnosis of acute abdominal pain. Recently this system was subjected to a stringent test under the auspices of the DHSS involving eight hospitals and 16,737 patients.[7] In this system the doctor who first saw each patient in hospital filled out a detailed questionnaire about the patient's symptoms and physical signs. These data were then entered into a small desk-top computer, which compared the data with those from 6000 other patients, and produced a diagnostic 'prediction' concerning the common causes of acute abdominal pain (Figure 11.2 and Table 11.2). This was then made available to the doctor managing the patient, who then made a decision about treatment.

Figure 11.2: Abdominal pain chart

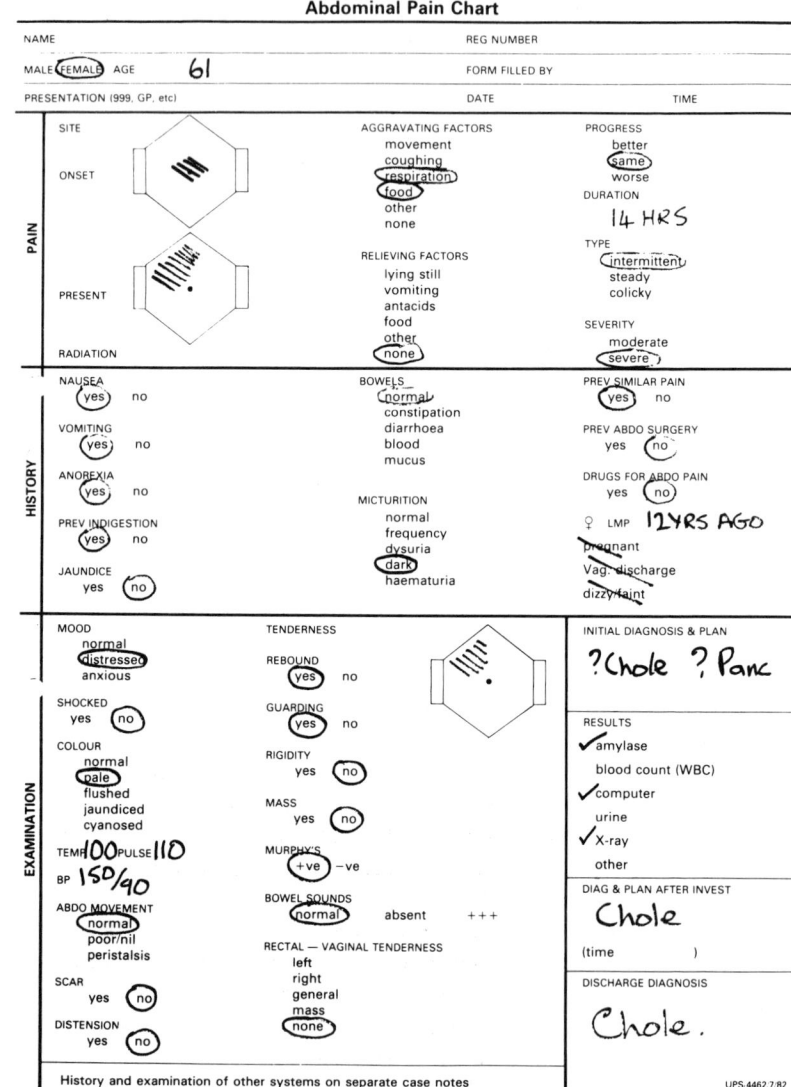

Table 11.2: Acute abdominal pain program

Computer user	:M. Chan
Date	:10th March 1987
Patient ident.	:54321
Status	:research assistant
Data collected by	:cons

User accepts clinical judgement must take precedence

HISTORY	:female
	age 60–69
	pain onset CENTRAL
	pain now RUQ
	aggrav by RESPIRATION
	aggrav by FOOD
	NO relief factors
	NO change
	pain 12–23 HRS
	INTERMITTENT now
	SEVERE
	NAUSEA
	VOMITING
	ANOREXIA
	previous INDIGESTION
	NO jaundice
	bowels NORMAL
	OTHER mict. symptoms
	previous SIMILAR PAIN
	NO prev ABDO SURGERY
	NOT taking DRUGS
EXAMINATION	:DISTRESSED
	PALE
	abdo movt. NORMAL
	NO SCAR
	NO distension
	tender RFQ
	REBOUND
	GUARDING
	NO rigidity
	NO swelling
	MURPHY +ve
	NORMAL bowel sounds
	NORMAL rectal exam
User diagnosis	:? Chole ? Panc
Management plan	:Investigate

COMPUTER DIAGNOSTIC PREDICTION	
Appendicitis	0
Divert. disease	0
Perforated Ulcer	0
Non specific	0
Cholecystitis	99
Obstruction	0
Pancreatitis	0
Renal Colic	0
Dyspepsia	0

Table 11.3: Summary of findings in recent DHSS trial of computer-aided decision support system for acute abdominal pain

	Baseline (4075 cases)	Trial period (12,662 cases)
Initial diagnostic accuracy	45.6%	65.3%
Post-investigation diagnostic accuracy	57.9%	74.2%
Percentage NSAP patients admitted from A/E	40.9%	26.3%
Percentage NSAP patients reattended A/E	7.4%	1.5%
Percentage NSAP patients operated on	9.5%	5.6%
Perforated appendicitis rate	23.7%	11.6%
Annual saving		
Negative laparotomies	—	139 p.a.
NSAP bed-nights	—	3387 p.a.
Appendicitis bed-nights	—	871 p.a.
Bad management errors	0.9%	0.2%
Death	1.2%	0.92%

Data from ref. 7

The results of adopting this procedure are shown in Table 11.3. From this study it is quite clear that the advent of the computer-aided system was associated with significant improvements in initial diagnosis, and also (interestingly) in diagnosis after investigation, since there seemed to be a 'knock-on' effect throughout the surgical team. There was also an improvement in decision-making — since negative laparotomy rates and perforation rates for appendicitis patients fell simultaneously, as did the mortality rate. Of comfort to the DHSS sponsoring the project, a total of 8000 bed-nights were saved, as were resources valued at around £700,000 in the eight hospitals.

This is most gratifying and encouraging. However, the study also made quite clear that not all of this improvement was due to the computer feedback. Around half of it was due to the clarification of terminology and discipline in data collection which took place even *before* the use of the computer. The evidence for this is simple: when doctors were given agreed data collection forms, and used them *without* the computer, they improved their diagnostic accuracy by 10 per cent.

RESIDUAL PROBLEMS

We have dealt in some detail with one specific system in order to demonstrate that there are indeed benefits to be obtained by the sensible use of computer systems in the clinical diagnostic process. But a number of further questions are raised by this system; pertinent questions which need to be answered before one can decide whether to adopt this technology or not.

Technical questions

Actually, these are simplest of all. What hardware should be used? What language should programs be written in? and so on. These are not problems which should concern the doctor so much as the computer scientist. In any case, the type of program designed to run the abdominal pain system is so simple that it can be, and has been, implemented on a pocket calculator. (Such implementation is not recommended, since it misses some of the useful computer educational functions, but the fact that it can be done illustrates that hardware and software problems are not the most pressing difficulties preventing implementation.)

The technical problems which remain are more logistic than technical. Even given the results set out in Table 11.3, it remains far from clear what is the best method of implementing such systems. Should hospitals/practices have their own computer systems with dedicated 'chips' for each clinical diagnostic area plugged into the back? Or should such systems be operated more centrally with GPs and/or hospitals 'ringing in' data to a central unit? To many people such questions may seem mundane; but they are quite vital to the sensible use of even the most promising system, and it has to be said that we have totally failed to tackle such important questions in this country at the time of writing.

Medical questions

These are far less simple, as might be expected. The first, and most obvious, pair of questions are: will such a system work in general practice and will it work for other clinical areas of medicine?

Many computer people totally fail to understand the great gulf fixed between hospital practice (where patients tend to present with 'well-packaged' problems), and general practice (where the nature of a patient's problem is often far more obscure). Thus the system outlined above might well prove totally inappropriate in general practice, partly because in hospital patients are usually seen far later in their illness, and in general practice the computer 'trained' to deal with hospital cases might need a completely new data set to work with.

Nevertheless, a number of systems have been tested in general practice, and have appeared to give promise. At least two of these have concerned dyspepsia: the Glasgow system already described, and a system tested in Yorkshire.[9,11,12] In this latter study a nursing sister or medical secretary interviewed patients with dyspepsia in health centres, and if the resultant data indicated upon computer analysis that the patient had a better than 10 per cent chance of cancer, the patient was referred for high technology. In both urban[11] and rural[12] GP environments this resulted in a stream of cases with cancer being identified and rapidly treated.

But perhaps the biggest medical problem which remains is that concerning terminology. In the clinical areas discussed (acute abdominal pain and dyspepsia), one of the principal benefits has been the derivation of an agreed, clarified terminology; and the fact has to be faced that for many areas of clinical medicine relevant to general practice, such agreed terminology does not exist (back pain is a good example of such an area).

In a sense this is both an opportunity and a challenge, since one major role which might be suggested for the practising clinician might well be to become involved in the development of such terminology. Even if one never subsequently went near a computer, all the evidence suggests that the development of agreed, clarified terminology is likely to be beneficial — it allows us to talk to each other even if we don't wish to talk to computers. Such considerations illustrate incidentally the value of information science as opposed to information technology in clinical medicine.

Ethical questions

The prospect of using computers in clinical diagnosis raises some interesting questions of an ethical nature. These are discussed more fully elsewhere,[13] but some brief remarks may be appropriate.

Ethical considerations are usually subdivided into questions relating to beneficence, non-malificence, autonomy and justice. In this instance we have already dealt at some length with the first two (systems should show beneficence, otherwise they should not be used, which implies careful *evaluation*; and non-maliﬁcence, so that they do not harm patients, which implies a *subordinate* role for the computer). The latter two problems, however, are much more complex, and deserve special mention.

Autonomy is perhaps the key problem — principally the autonomy of the doctor using the system. Clinical freedom, as Hampton reminds us, 'is dead. . . . It was at worst a cloak for incompetence'.[14] This is a slightly harsh judgement, for no-one is seriously suggesting that a doctor's autonomy should be entirely subjugated to that of an automated system. It is, however, worth pointing out that clinical freedom — in the sense that the doctor can do whatever he or she wishes with complete impunity — probably *is* dead in this day and age. It is also worth pointing out that there is a great difference between an obligation slavishly to do what the computer says (which is probably rather silly), and an obligation to analyse symptoms thoroughly and to take a computer system's prediction into account when making a final judgement (which probably once more places the computer in the same position as an X-ray or blood test. One might not be pilloried for over-ruling a 'normal' ECG; but equally, one might be thought at fault if one had not performed the test in the first place.)

Finally, it is worth pointing out that 'clinical freedom', in the sense of a God-given right, never existed at all. Clinical freedom is conferred by society upon a doctor in the expectation that such freedom will be used to the benefit of each individual patient. It implies an obligation upon the doctor to make the best judgement he can about each patient, using whatever additional sources of help he needs and can acquire; and if that includes (*inter alia*) a computer prediction, then so be it.

But what happens when the prediction or the doctor, or both, are wrong? Surely justice demands that someone is to blame?

First, we need to distinguish between 'strict' liability, which implies that whenever a patient doesn't get better, someone is at fault, and 'product' liability, which implies that the doctor and/or the system have to be seen to make an error before any form of judicial compensation is called for.[15] In the UK we have opted in the main for the latter; a recent ruling suggested that a doctor could not be held negligent if he or she had followed a course of action which a group of his peers, respected and respectable, skilled and experienced, would have done in the same situation. The computer (by the same token) could only be held at fault if it had failed to perform in the manner in which the doctor was entitled to expect that it would.

Bearing in mind the ancillary role already discussed for the computer, this does not pose too many immediate problems. There are, however, some consequential arguments which need to be explored. First, this raises yet again the question of evaluation. The computer system, like any other special investigation, needs to have a comprehensive track record; and the doctor using it needs to know what this is. The doctor needs to know, for example, whether the computer is basing its prediction upon comparison with real-life patients or upon the 'expert thoughts' of a possibly fallible doctor. The doctor also needs to know the track record of the computer in a given situation (for how else can the computer prediction be put properly into an overall context by the doctor?).

Second, and perhaps more positively, the computer system may be seen as protecting the doctor in the event of an unfortunate consequence of treatment. For in the type of system outlined above,[7] where the framework has been constructed by over 200 doctors working in concert, in following the computer's *modus operandi* the individual doctor is clearly adopting a framework for diagnosis adopted by a group of doctors, skilled and respected. As such it becomes that much easier for a doctor to demonstrate that, in this instance, proper agreed practice *was* followed; and it becomes that much more difficult to demonstrate that a doctor has been negligent simply because the patient failed to get better.

CONCLUSIONS

From the various arguments set out above, certain conclusions can be drawn, and these may now be itemised for clarity.

1. There is really no point talking about *when* computers will be able to mimic diagnosis, or assist a doctor in deciding what is wrong with a patient. In the sense described above, they already can do so.

2. There is also no doubt from recent studies that doctors aided by computers have performed better than those who were not so aided; both in the sense that diagnostic performance was improved, and also in the sense that patient care improved, and scarce resources were saved to be used elsewhere.

3. At the moment, however, the computer is only of proven benefit in certain very restricted areas of medicine. Computers cannot 'do diagnosis'. They can only assist the doctor once the doctor has elicited the information from the patient, and decided what the patient's main problem area is.

4. Unfortunately, the latter activity is of paramount importance in general practice. This implies that diagnostic computers may be used sooner and more widely in hospitals (where the problem is more frequently clear-cut) than in general practice (where the problem is more frequently somewhat nebulous until clarified by the GP).

5. Nevertheless, we may expect to see quite a number of systems dealing with specific areas of medicine over the next few years. The GP should pay particular attention, in deciding whether to use such systems, to their evaluation. Systems which are not thoroughly evaluated are intrinsically dangerous and should be avoided.

6. Particularly important — perhaps the main contribution to date of computer technology in clinical medicine — has been the re-emphasis which it places upon traditional clinical virtues such as careful history-taking. If the computer does no more than remind us (because of its own inherent simplicity) that we need to phrase our questions to the patient carefully, and listen carefully to the patient's story before flying to high technology, then it will have been well worth having in the long run!

REFERENCES

1. Taylor, T.R. (1970) Computers in medicine in the decade of the 1970s. *Scottish Medical Journal*, *15*, 353
2. de Dombal, F.T. (1979) Picking the best tests in acute abdominal pain. *Journal of the Royal College of Physicians*, London, *13*, 203
3. Gill, P.W., Leaper, D.J. and Guillou, P.J. (1973) Observer variation in clinical diagnosis. A computer-aided assessment of its magnitude and importance in 552 patients with abdominal pain. *Methods of Information in Medicine*, *12*, 108
4. Leaper, D.J., Gill, P.W. and Staniland, J.R. (1973) Clinical diagnostic process: an analysis. *British Medical Journal*, *3*, 569
5. MacAdam, D.B. (1979) A study in general practice of the symptoms and delay patterns in the diagnosis of gastrointestinal cancer. *Journal of the Royal College of General Practitioners*, *29*, 723

6. Dixon, R.H. and Laszlo, J. (1974) Utilisation of clinical chemistry services by medical house staff. *Archives of Internal Medicine*, *134*, 1064

7. Adams, I.D., Chan, M. and Clifford, P.C. (1986) Computer-aided diagnosis of acute abdominal pain: a multi-centre study. *British Medical Journal*, *293*, 800

8. Mueller, B.A., Daling, J.R. and Moore, D.E. (1986) Appendectomy and the risk of tubal infertility. *New England Journal of Medicine*, *315*, 1506

9. Knill Jones, R.P. (1985) A formal approach to symptoms in dyspepsia. *Clinics in Gastroenterology*, *14*, 517

10. de Dombal, F.T. and Hall, R. (1979) The evaluation of medical care to the clinician's point of view. Can we trust our own assessments. In: Alperovitch, A., de Dombal, F.T., Gremy, F. (eds), *Measuring the efficacy of medical care*. Proceedings of IFIP Working Conference, Bordeaux. North Holland, Amsterdam

11. Clamp, S.E. and Wenham, J.S. (1984) Interviewing by paramedics with computer analysis: Gastro-intestinal cancer. In: Rozen, P. and de Dombal, F.T. (eds), *Frontiers of gastro-intestinal research: computer aids in gastroenterology*. S. Karger AG, Basel, Switzerland, p. 186

12. Davenport, P.M., Morgan, A.G. and Darnborough, A. (1985) Can preliminary screening of dyspeptic patients allow more effective use of investigational techniques. *British Medical Journal*, *290*, 217

13. de Dombal, F.T. (1987) Ethical considerations concerning computers in medicine in the 1980s. *Journal of Medical Ethics* (in press)

14. Hampton, J.R. (1983) The end of clinical freedom. *British Medical Journal*, *287*, 1237

15. Dyer, C. (1986) Product liability comes closer. *British Medical Journal*, *293*, 1489

12

Aids to Clinical Management

Bob Jones

Computer systems as yet offer little in the way of information for the management of individual patients within the consultation. The main uses of computers in the UK are related to office procedures or to call/recall of populations.[1] Elsewhere billing and financial management take pride of place. However, this situation is likely to change. In a recent survey of computerised UK practices[2] among 514 completed questionnaires 'use during the consultation' came second in priority on the list of 21 suggestions which the practices would most like to see developed.

Waiting in the wings for this change to take place are a number of projects concerned with individual patient management which need a terminal in the consulting room to be fully effective. Some of these developments are being tested in a hospital environment. Others are being piloted by Health Authorities or by computer practices. Their significance as regards patient management will be described in this chapter.

FLAGGING AND REMINDERS

Flags such as coloured labels to indicate important diseases, and reminders of dates when preventive procedures are due to be carried out, are relatively common on manual records. This idea has been incorporated and developed for use in medical computer systems, particularly in America. At the Regenstrief Institute in Indianapolis an automated medical record (RMIS) for use in outpatients has been steadily developed over a number of years.[3] Duke University Medical Centre[4] and the Massachusetts General Hospital[5] have also been active in this field, producing a number of systems (TMR and COSTAR) which are marketed commercially. Features which most of these systems have in common include:

(1) the ability to display problem lists and active prescriptions;

(2) the ability to flag abnormal results of examinations or of investigations (such as blood tests or X-rays) in such a way that it would be difficult for the clinician to overlook them;

(3) reminders of actions which should be considered by the clinician as a consequence of a diagnosis, test result, or treatment.

Flags

These are a particular feature of the Regenstrief Medical Information System. Used to highlight abnormal features found on examining the patient or abnormal results of investigations (e.g. blood tests or X-rays) they are commonly linked to reminders.

Reminders

When a patient is seen at a clinic in the Wishard Memorial Hospital (which is associated with the Regenstrief Institute) the computer-produced encounter form, which is available for each consultation, is accompanied by a 'reminder report' which details the reminders associated with that patient. Examples of reminders quoted by McDonald et al[3] include:

(1) for people whose weight is more than 130 per cent of ideal weight, consider a diet;

(2) for people on diuretics or potassium supplements an annual check on serum potassium level may be advisable;

(3) for people who have had a myocardial infarct consider beta-blockers to prevent sudden death;

(4) people with chronic airways disease should be immunised against influenza in the autumn.

These reminders are based on 'rules' which have been agreed among themselves by the clinicians practising in the Wishard Memorial Hospital. A total of 1491 rules were formulated during consideration

Figure 12.1: Example of a reminder report

19-Mar-86 "ENTRY CTL:CO6"

Please return to Regenstrief Institute, do not chart.

TIDBITS FROM THE COMPUTER

These suggestions are based on incomplete data; your judgement should take precedence.

SAMPLE, PATIENT #9999999-7 AGE:6 SEX:M
RACE:W
PHONE: 234-5678
Scheduled to MCDONALD, CLEMENT on 25-Dec-86 at 01:30 PM (O)

Consider yearly screen of stool for occult blood to monitor GI tract bleeding risk in patient with BULB DEFORMED

Consider getting chest x-ray every 2 years to follow CARDIOMEGALY reported on 01-Nov-80.

Consider use of nystatin or miconazole to treat monilia, diagnosed on 23-SEP-85.

---

of the actions which *should* be undertaken in different clinical situations. From these rules 751 reminder messages were generated. An example of a reminder report is shown in Figure 12.1.

PROTOCOLS AND FLOWSHEETS

Protocols for the management of people with specific diseases, based on practice policies, are rare. Most general practitioners working in partnerships have difficulty in agreeing protocols and then acting on them. There are also practical difficulties in storing a number of flowsheets in a Lloyd-George medical record envelope.

Figure 12.2: Basic drug information provided on sophisticated computer systems

Pack size 500			DHSS approved				Cost of 500 ml = £4.37	
Date	Pharma-ceutical name	Form	Strength	Dosage	Days	Qty	Op Rp	Is Comm.
19.3.87	GAVISCON	LIQ	00	PRN	30	1	6	4

Another feature which the American medical computer systems previously mentioned have in common is that when a specific diagnosis is established for a patient this triggers the production of a flowsheet appropriate to the particular disease or condition. A renal disease flowsheet might contain the results of previous examinations of the urine, the blood for urea creatinine and electrolytes, the weight and blood pressure. One for thyroid disease could include blood tests for T4, TSH, presence or absence of tremor and eye signs, weight, blood pressure. The tests, clinical examination and timing of review consultations can be arranged in such a way as to remind the clinician of currently accepted management.

DRUG INFORMATION

In simple computer systems it is rare for information about drugs, their interactions or side-effects, to be available. In more sophisticated systems basic information (see Figure 12.2) is provided when a drug is to be prescribed.

This background information could clearly be expanded. Preece et al[6] have shown one way in which this could be done, describing the development of a 'drug intelligence package'. Such packages are now commercially available. Further developments are in the pipeline. For example, when a general practitioner wishes to prescribe a fresh drug for a patient it is technically possible to test for contraindication against any part of that patient's record, against drugs already being taken (e.g. anticoagulants), against conditions such as asthma or pregnancy — as well as showing price, pack size and possible side-effects. The usefulness of this facility also depends on the presence of a terminal in the consulting room.

Shared with the patient

In most consultations agreement between patient and doctor on management is reached without too much difficulty: whether to rest or be active, to go to work or stay at home, to continue to eat normally or partake of a special diet, are not questions which are complicated or which need support from outside or access to data banks. During other consultations more complex management problems arise. The complexity may be due to the subject matter, or to the volume of information which has to be exchanged. For someone who has been found to have a hiatus hernia, rheumatoid arthritis or diabetes, both the content of the information and the amount are difficult to encompass verbally within a normal consultation. Printed information is available in the form of leaflets or books but the motivation of many practitioners to maintain an up-to-date comprehensive stock of literature is blunted by the multiplicity of sources and the variable quality of the products; as well as by the saturation effect of volumes of printed material thumping on the doormat daily.

In Chapter 15 Neil Carson describes educational material for patients which is currently being designed and piloted in Australia. In the USA a system for use with microcomputers, which provides patient information for paediatric problems, is currently being marketed. The availability of a comprehensive range of management information for a whole range of diseases and complaints within one computer package is a real prospect in the near future. Such information will be able to be viewed or printed, to be seen by the doctor and patient together, to be viewed by the patient at a separate terminal, or to be taken home in printed form.

THE SMART CARD

This is the name given to a plastic card similar to a credit card, on which a memory bank has been imprinted. In France, where the main development has taken place, these cards have mainly been used for financial transactions. Increase in the limited capacity of the card (from 8k to 32k in 1987, with further increases in the pipeline) means that the possibility of medical use is being considered. Several simple programs already exist, providing a limited portable medical record. Clearly there is immense scope for development. The projection is that within three years cards no bigger than a credit card will be able to carry all information which is normally present in a patient's practice record together with a proportion of his or her hospital record. The cards will be 'read' through an electronic reader to a microcomputer and shown on the screen. In current French medical applications access depends on a two-key system — with the patient having a personal identity number (PIN) and the physician having his/her own 'access' card with coded number. Both access keys are needed at the same time to enable the reader to function. In the USA Blue Cross and Blue Shield of Maryland is currently promoting a credit card-sized 'Life Card' for the storage of X-rays and results of laboratory investigations.

Clearly there are all sorts of matters besides confidentiality and access to be considered before use of these cards as a personal portable medical record within the NHS becomes the norm, but the technology is there and in use. Yet another source of information for use in management of individual patients is imminent.

FROM OUTSIDE THE PRACTICE

The advent of electronic communication between systems outside the practice and the practice system is being pioneered in the UK by Health Net. British Telecom and a Health Authority are co-operating to pilot its use within a health district. The concept of Health Net is simple. Messages are transmitted from one terminal (e.g. in a hospital, pathological laboratory, ambulance station) to another terminal (e.g. in a practice or nurse station or social worker's office) by telephone line. Transmission between terminals is possible in both directions.

Development of this concept has major implications for management of individual patients within general practice.

For *clinical management* the automatic transfer of results and reports from hospital to practice implies that such information could either be printed in the practice or could, if appropriate, be entered directly into the patient's record in a structured fashion. Information for management would be quickly and clearly available.

Moreover, the protocols of local consultants for specific conditions could be made available to practitioners through this link — at what age the surgeon would like to see a boy with an undescended testicle in outpatients, what criteria would the orthopaedic surgeon use in deciding when to carry out a total hip replacement on a person with an arthritic hip, what investigations would the gastroenterologist like done before he sees the patient?

For *non-clinical management* the availability of electronic communication would enable the practitioner to be aware during the consultation of the bed states and outpatient waiting times of the local hospitals, of the vacancies, facilities and cost of local residential and nursing homes, of the availability of home helps or meals-on-wheels. Moreover services could be requested through such a link directly to the agencies concerned.

MANAGEMENT FEEDBACK

The introduction of reminders, the availability of flowsheets, of drug information and of other management information appropriate to individual patients will provide a structure against which a practitioner can compare his actions or lack of action. Until now automatic feedback such as this has been rare in general practice. It is provided by the maternity co-operation card, which indicates what has been done or not done; whether, for example, the patient has been weighed or not on her last three visits.

Depending on the introduction of terminals into the consulting room, and on agreement over protocols (either within a practice, locally or nationally), the prospect is that automatic feedback about clinical management behaviour will become available for individual doctors treating patients with a large range of conditions. Experience has shown[7] that availability of such information has a profound effect on doctor behaviour.

SUMMARY

The simplest way to summarise how computers will affect clinical management by general practitioners within the foreseeable future is to describe the scenario when a man aged 55 returns to his general practitioner for the result of a fasting blood sugar, his original complaint the day before having been of thirst and nocturia, his midmorning urine having shown 1 per cent glucose.

When he enters the consulting room the practitioner is already looking at his computer summary on the screen. The result of the fasting blood sugar, transmitted by Health Net, is blinking at them both. As the practitioner explains the significance of this result he enters DIAB on the keyboard, at which a 'menu' appears enquiring whether he wishes a diabetic flowsheet, management protocol, hospital policy, drug information about drugs used in diabetes, or management/educational material. The computer is 'aware' of the age–sex previous history and present medication of the patient. All the information produced under each 'menu heading' will take account of these facts.

After discussing the main issues patient and doctor decide that the treatment will be by diet and glibenclamide initially, that the patient will go into the next room, view the educational material and have printed those items he wishes to mull over at home. His prescription (having been checked) will be issued and accompanied by a note of the address of the Diabetic Association, a sheet for recording the results of his urine tests and a diet sheet. His next appointment with the practice nurse or doctor will have been made by the time he leaves the room. All the relevant information will have been entered on his practice record and his 'smart card' by one simple entry of each fact.

In this instance as described the practitioner will have used but a fraction of the management information which is available under 'Diabetes'.

Although the technology is available to turn this scenario into reality for general practice now, it will be the attitudes of practitioners, finance and the double pressures from government and consumer which will determine the speed at which it occurs.

REFERENCES

1. Fitter, M.J., Garber, J.R., Herzmark, G.A., Robinson, D. and Jones, R.V.H. (1986) *A Prescription for Change*. HMSO, London
2. DHSS/NHS Information Technology Branch (1987) *Survey of Computerized Practices*. Crown copyright
3. McDonald, C.J., Hai, S.L., Smith, D.M., Tierney, W.M., Cohen, S.J., Weinberger, M. and McCabe, G.P. (1984) Reminders to physicians from an introspective medical record: a two year randomized trial. *Annals of Internal Medicine*, *100*, 130–8
4. Stead, W.W., Garrett, L.E. and Hammond, W.E. (1983) Practicing nephrology with a computerized medical record. *Kidney International*, *24*, 446–54
5. Barnett, G.O. (1984) The application of computer based medical record systems in ambulatory practice. *New England Journal of Medicine*, *310*, 1643–50
6. Preece, J.F., Ashford, J.R. and Hunt, R.G. (1984) Writing all prescriptions by computer. *Journal of the Royal College of General Practitioners*, *34*, 655–7
7. McDonald, C.J. (1976) Protocol-based computer reminders, the quality of care and the non-perfectability of man. *New England Journal of Medicine*, *295*, 1351–5

13

Artificial Intelligence

John Fox, Andrzej Glowinski and Michael O'Neil

INTRODUCTION: ARTIFICIAL INTELLIGENCE AND KNOWLEDGE ENGINEERING

Artificial intelligence (AI) appeared about 1965 when it was seen as a science which was concerned with understanding the principles of 'intelligence' rather than a kind of computer engineering. The scope of AI research was wide. It included perception (understanding the mechanisms of vision and hearing), understanding language (the spoken and written word), decision-making, problem-solving, learning and so on. In some areas progress was rapid, if controversial, but few people expected the next major development — the appearance of practical 'knowledge-based' systems.

By 1975 a number of AI systems had been developed that appeared to solve difficult practical problems in medicine, science and engineering. It was not that intelligence was now understood, but that symbolic computing techniques had been developed which could be applied to specialist problems at a level which would require considerable human expertise. The practical subject that emerged from this came to be called 'knowledge engineering', which can be thought of as the design of computer systems able to cope with tasks which would require intelligence if carried out by people, and which exploit, in part, human understanding of the tasks.

AI has always been controversial. One of the reasons for this is that there are few subjects which AI has tackled which other disciplines have not previously attacked. Table 13.1 summarises these topics and their earlier counterparts. However, the key technical ideas of the AI approach are very different from the earlier, algorithmic, often highly mathematical computer techniques.

157

Table 13.1: AI and other disciplines compared

Artificial intelligence	'Conventional' information engineering
Problem-solving/inference	Statistical decision analysis
Language understanding	Machine translation
Speech understanding	Word recognition
Visual image interpretation	Pattern recognition
Object manipulation	Robots
Learning	Adaptive control theory

The concept which cuts across much of AI, and which is central to knowledge-based systems, is the explicit representation and use of knowledge.

We can illustrate this by comparing the knowledge-based approach with the traditional mathematical approach to computer-assisted diagnosis. For more than 20 years statisticians and others have developed mathematical methods of decision-making, personnel selection, resource planning and so on. This was often done with great success, and there are a number of well-known examples in medicine. The basic concept is quite simple. Suppose a patient presents with certain symptoms and we wish to analyse these symptoms and decide upon a probable diagnosis. To do this we would typically use a data base containing a set of numerical parameters, such as conditional probabilities which represent the likelihood of particular symptoms occurring with particular diseases. Then some mathematical procedure, such as Bayes' rule for calculating probabilities, uses this data base to calculate the mathematical likelihood of each possible diagnosis for the patient, given his or her specific symptoms.

Knowledge-based systems have also been developed for diagnostic and other decisions, but their superficial similarity to the traditional mathematical methods is deceptive. Knowledge-based systems emphasise qualitative, logical reasoning rather than quantitative calculation. Logical inference requires logical data so the data base of an expert system does not contain numbers exclusively, and may not contain numbers at all. We call this material the 'knowledge base'.

The key feature of a knowledge base is that its contents are not abstract symbols like conditional probabilities or other numbers. Probabilities record the magnitude of a relationship, like the relationship between a symptom and a disease, but not its 'meaning'.

Knowledge-based systems for assisting decision-making frequently exploit large quantities of information about a subject or 'domain' such as medicine, making its meaning as explicit and complete as possible rather than reducing it to an abstract form. They also make extensive use of information about the way these facts are to be used, commonly expressed as 'rules of thumb' and sometimes informally referred to as 'knowhow'.

Facts and rules can be used to represent a wide range of medical knowledge, ranging from knowledge about causes, symptoms and treatments of diseases, the cost, invasiveness and informativeness of investigations, the indications, contraindications and side-effects of drugs and so on. The knowledge-based approach also permits us to take advantage of taxonomic information, as in the taxonomy of drugs and classifications of diseases, similar to taxonomies used to classify living organisms into species, families and genera. This factual information can be manipulated by conventional programs or by 'if . . . then . . . rules'. Although these rules seem very simple they can represent a huge variety of problem-solving and decision-making techniques. In this chapter the history of the Oxford System of Medicine project is described in detail as an example of the way in which artificial intelligence may in future be used in the setting of general practice.

HISTORY OF THE PROJECT

The Biomedical Computing Unit of the Imperial Cancer Research Fund has an established programme of research into medical decision-making, and a special interest in computer systems for general practice. Effective screening, early detection, accurate diagnosis and management of cancer, can all benefit from computer technology, though only as an integrated part of general medical practice.

Oxford University Press is a major medical publisher, now also involved in electronic publishing. During 1985 the Press asked Peter Pritchard, a general practitioner and writer on practice management, to carry out a study into whether a new kind of medical information service, called the 'Oxford System of Medicine' (OSM), might be developed for use in the 1990s. The OSM would be a computerised information system designed to assist GPs in making a wide range of medical decisions — a clinical tool for doctors having to keep pace with the large and growing body of modern medical knowledge. It was clear that development of the OSM would require considerable resources; even so, it was uncertain whether a practical design was within the present state of the art.

Dr Pritchard's study reported[1] that the OSM might be possible, and the ICRF and OUP agreed to collaborate. Earlier work on interactive systems for clinical decision support[2] on the design of the user interface and the clinical impact of such systems[3,4] and the establishment of a design for a knowledge-based general practice information system[5,6] provided the starting point for the exercise.

THE PROTOTYPE CONCEPT

The concept of the OSM is illustrated in Figure 13.1. A small personal computer on the doctor's desk (independent or linked to other machines in the practice) is immediately to hand during a patient consultation. The OSM must provide information in a variety of ways. Frequently, doctors may only require a quick, convenient way of getting access to information — some detail about a patient, drug, disease, investigation or local service. Sometimes, however, the doctor may find it useful to have assistance in making a specific diagnostic or management decision. In this circumstance the computer must be able to automatically locate any information from both the medical knowledge and patient record, however obscure, which could be relevant to the decision. Occasionally the doctor may even value a 'second opinion': What is the most plausible diagnosis? What would be the best treatment or investigation? How might the treatment or investigative procedure be planned?

AIMS OF THE PILOT PROJECT

The OSM pilot project explored the practical and theoretical possibility of developing a system with these characteristics. The six-month study started with three specific aims:

(1) To assess whether an OSM is technically feasible and suitable for development or whether it is still a distant goal requiring further research.

(2) To explore the facilities that might be needed for an OSM to have practical value to general practitioners and to develop

Figure 13.1

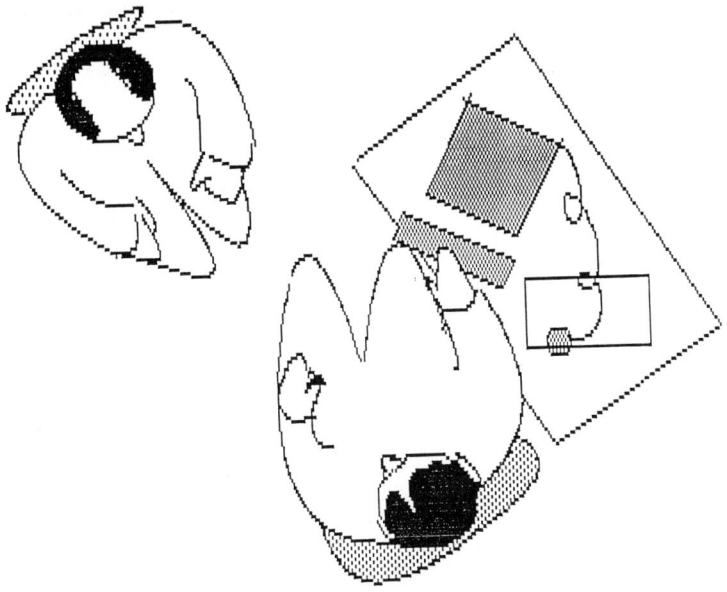

a prototype incorporating some of these facilities.

(3) To consider whether the Oxford System of Medicine could be designed in such a way that a routine procedure could be established for electronic publication of medical knowledge to high medical and technical standards.

THE PROTOTYPE DESIGN

Figure 13.2 illustrates the user's view of the prototype. This layout has three main areas. At the top are four control panels, labelled 'information', 'assistance', 'synopsis' and 'explanation'. These provide menu-based access to four groups of facilities: access to information about patients, drugs, diseases, investigations and treatments; an 'assistant' for decision-making; various facilities for summarising and reviewing the case; explanations of questions, conclusions and so on. Other facilities would be needed in a mature system. The large centre panel is used for presenting information to

Figure 13.2

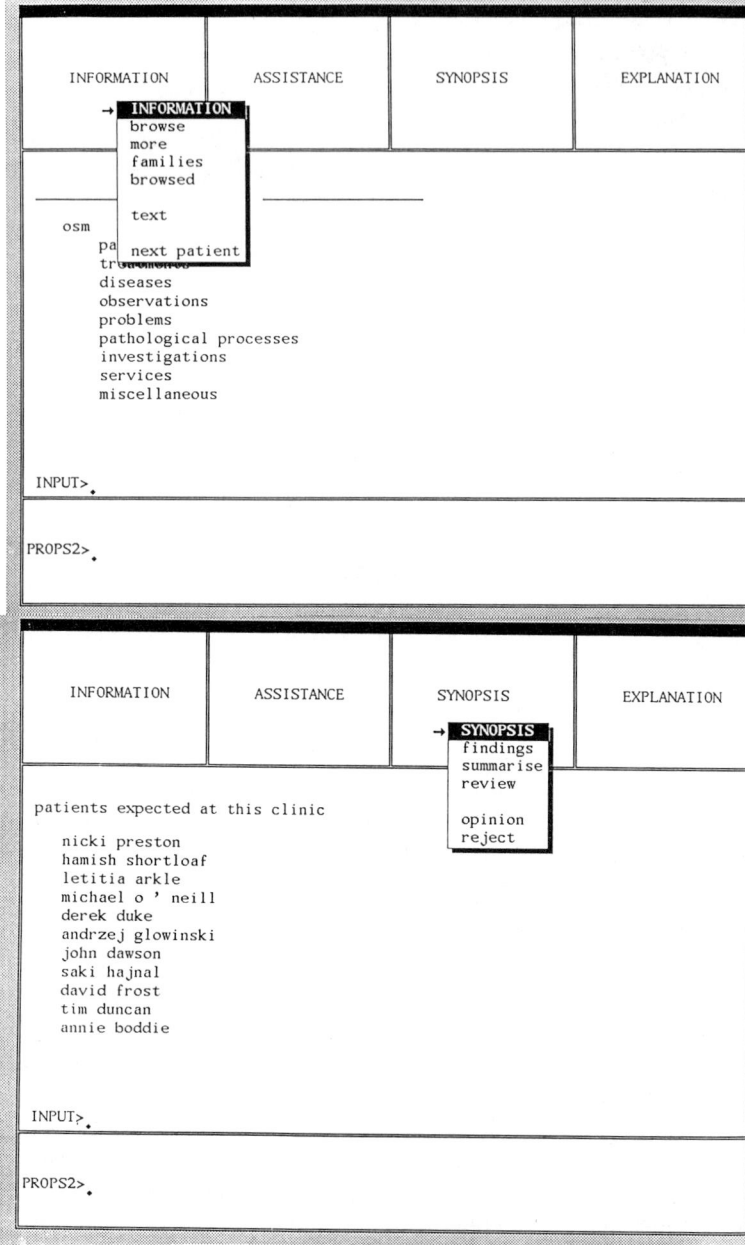

```
┌─────────────┬─────────────┬─────────────┬─────────────┐
│ INFORMATION │ ASSISTANCE  │  SYNOPSIS   │ EXPLANATION │
│             │           → │ ASSISTANCE  │             │
│             │             │ classify    │             │
│             │             │ investigate │             │
│ patients expected at th│ treat       │             │
│                       │ prescribe   │             │
│    nicki preston      │             │             │
│    hamish shortloaf   │ include     │             │
│    letitia arkle      │ exclude     │             │
│    michael o'neill                                  │
│    derek duke                                       │
│    andrzej glowinski                                │
│    john dawson                                      │
│    saki hajnal                                      │
│    david frost                                      │
│    tim duncan                                       │
│    annie boddie                                     │
│                                                     │
│ INPUT>.                                             │
├─────────────────────────────────────────────────────┤
│ PROPS2>.                                            │
└─────────────────────────────────────────────────────┘
```

```
┌─────────────┬─────────────┬─────────────┬─────────────┐
│ INFORMATION │ ASSISTANCE  │  SYNOPSIS   │ EXPLANATION │
│             │             │             │ → EXPLANATION│
│             │             │             │   question  │
│             │             │             │   method    │
│             │             │             │   reasoning │
│ ──────────────── osm ────────────────               │
│  osm                                                │
│     patients                                        │
│     treatments                                      │
│     diseases                                        │
│     observations                                    │
│     problems                                        │
│     pathological processes                          │
│     investigations                                  │
│     services                                        │
│     miscellaneous                                   │
│                                                     │
│ INPUT>.                                             │
├─────────────────────────────────────────────────────┤
│ PROPS2>.                                            │
└─────────────────────────────────────────────────────┘
```

Figure 13.3

| INFORMATION | ASSISTANCE | SYNOPSIS | EXPLANATION |

```
                      drugs
     drugs
         anaesthetic drugs
         anti infective drugs
         antimalignancy drugs
         cardiovascular drugs
         central nervous system drugs
         dermatological drugs
         endocrine drugs
         gastrointestinal drugs
         immunological drugs
         immunosuppressive drugs
         musculoskeletal drugs
                                              (continued..)
INPUT>

PROPS2>
```

| INFORMATION | ASSISTANCE | SYNOPSIS | EXPLANATION |

```
                      cimetidine
     cimetidine
         tagamet
         contraindications
         duration
         formulations
         injection
         label
         tablet
         dose per day
         maximum duration
         maximum dose per day
                                              (continued..)
INPUT>

PROPS2>
```

| INFORMATION | ASSISTANCE | SYNOPSIS | EXPLANATION |

———————— h2 receptor blocking drugs ————————

h2 receptor blocking drugs
    cimetidine
    ranitidine

INPUT>

PROPS2>

| INFORMATION | ASSISTANCE | SYNOPSIS | EXPLANATION |

———————— contraindications ————————

antacids
anticoagulants
benzodiazepine hypnotics
carbamazepine
clonazepam
flecanide
impaired hepatic function
impaired renal function
ketoconazole
labetalol
lignocaine
metronidazole
                                                (continued..)

INPUT>

PROPS2>

Figure 13.4

INFORMATION	ASSISTANCE	SYNOPSIS	EXPLANATION

```
                         _____  ASSISTANCE
                                           classify
                                           investigate
                        strong narcotics   treat
                                         ▶ prescribe
    strong narcotics
        buprenorphine                      include
        dextromoramide                     exclude
        diamorphine
        dipipanone
        levonorphanol
        meptazinol
        methadone
        morphine
        nalbuphine
        papaveretum
        pethidine
                                                          (continued..)

INPUT>.

PROPS2>.
```

INFORMATION	ASSISTANCE	SYNOPSIS	EXPLANATION

```
choose any of the following factors - finish with ' ok '

    age group is child
    asthma
    liver failure
    parenteral route needed
    respiratory depression
    terminal care




INPUT>.

PROPS2>.
```

| INFORMATION | ASSISTANCE | SYNOPSIS | EXPLANATION |

```
_____ strong narcotics _____

  strong narcotics
     buprenorphine
     dextromoramide
     diamorphine
     dipipanone
     levonorphanol
     meptazinol
     methadone
     morphine
     nalbuphine
     papaveretum
     pethidine
                                              (continued..)
INPUT>
```

PROPS2>.

| INFORMATION | ASSISTANCE | SYNOPSIS | EXPLANATION |

```
prescription for morphine on 1 - 4 - 1919 for hamish shortloaf , age 54

    = = = warning - controlled drug - prescription must be handwritten = = =

    dose
              5  mg
    taken
              4  times a day
    duration
              7  days
    formulation
              elixir
    labels

                                                       (continued..)
INPUT>.
```

PROPS2>.

Figure 13.5

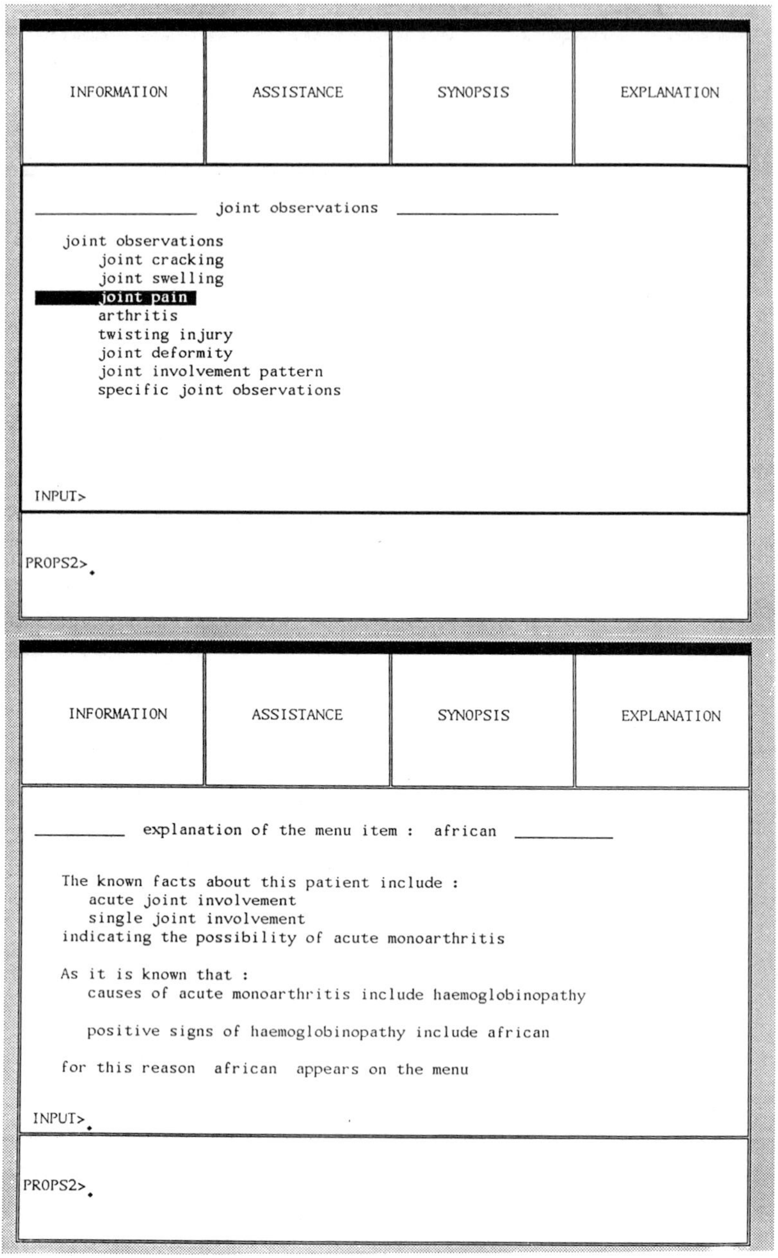

| INFORMATION | ASSISTANCE | SYNOPSIS | EXPLANATION |

─────────── joint observations ───────────

```
joint observations
   joint cracking
   joint swelling
   joint pain
   arthritis
   twisting injury
   joint deformity
   joint involvement pattern
   specific joint observations
```

INPUT>

PROPS2>.

| INFORMATION | ASSISTANCE | SYNOPSIS | EXPLANATION |

─────────── explanation of the menu item : african ───────────

The known facts about this patient include :
   acute joint involvement
   single joint involvement
indicating the possibility of acute monoarthritis

As it is known that :
   causes of acute monoarthritis include haemoglobinopathy

   positive signs of haemoglobinopathy include african

for this reason african appears on the menu

INPUT>.

PROPS2>.

| INFORMATION | ASSISTANCE | SYNOPSIS | EXPLANATION |

please select any of the following indicants - finish with ' ok '

   african
   anaemia
   bruising
   child
   chronic joint involvement
   distal interphalangeal joint arthritis
   first metarsophalangeal joint arthritis
   hyperuricaemia
   large joint arthritis
   multiple joint involvement
   proximal interphalangeal joint arthritis
   sacroiliitis

INPUT>.

PROPS2>.

| INFORMATION | ASSISTANCE | SYNOPSIS | EXPLANATION |

_____ summary of classifications _____(continued..)

   seronegative spondoarthritis
      confirmed positive signs   1
   haemophilia
   haemoglobinopathy
   psoriatic arthropathy
   ankylosing spondylitis
   reiters disease
      confirmed positive signs   4
   enteropathic arthritis
   behcets disease
   urethritis
   shigella dysentery

INPUT>.

PROPS2>.

the user, and for entering patient data using a mouse or other pointing device. The small bottom panel (which is optional) allows direct access to Props 2, the package used for development of the OSM prototype.[7]

Figure 13.3 illustrates the use of the OSM prototype with a simple sequence of screens produced while looking up prescribing information on the drug cimetidine. Figure 13.4 illustrates the use of the assistant, in this case to prescribe morphine. Figure 13.5 shows a slightly more complex use of the assistant in the classification (differential diagnosis) of joint pain.

THE USER INTERFACE

Ease of use and understanding are vital to the acceptability of computer systems, perhaps nowhere more so than in medicine. One of the contributions of early medical expert systems[8] was to emphasise the importance of good user interface design. In general practice time pressures and the unpredictable nature of the work make the design of the OSM's user interface particularly critical. To achieve acceptability several obvious requirements must be satisfied.

The first requirement is simplicity of operation. One of the most successful recent innovations in user-interface design is the combination of 'menu' and 'mouse'. In the OSM the mouse can be used to operate a menu, issue commands or enter an item of data by pointing at a word or phrase on the screen. Pressing a button mounted in the mouse confirms the selection.

The second requirement is conceptual simplicity. The facade in Figures 13.2–13.5 seems to be successful in that it is easy to grasp and physically simple to operate with few errors.* Many enhancements are possible, including graphics (e.g. for displaying blood pressure graphs), static and moving images from a laser disc (such as a rash or an abnormal gait). The added complexity of such enhancements could have disadvantages as well as advantages.

Of equal importance is the subtler requirement that the system be responsive to changing requirements as judged by the practitioner. The system should be controlled by the user, not vice-versa. Props

---

* The 'facade' seen by the user is easily altered to reflect different views of the OSM, without substantially altering the internal organisation or facilities. Other versions have had both simpler and more complicated facades.

2, in which the OSM prototype is implemented, permits any action at any time without intricate command protocols. This offers considerable freedom to the user. The OSM prototype extends this by providing a mechanism which allows interruption of any activity at any point simply by starting another process, returning to the suspended activity whenever desired. For instance, during diagnosis summaries or explanations of the current conclusions can be obtained, possible treatments considered or any topic 'looked up' (by invoking the information browser and pointing to the required topic with the mouse — see Figure 13.2) before resuming the interrupted diagnostic process. Since the OSM is intended for use in the clinical setting, where information requirements can be unpredictable and can change rapidly, we believe that at least this degree of flexibility is critical. The OSM must provide a range of information facilities. The prototype provides these but in an elective rather than dictatorial style.

Finally, the system can offer an 'opinion' on a diagnosis or suggest a prescription if — but only if — instructed to do so; even here the user can modify a suggested prescription, or reject a suggested diagnosis, or instruct the computer to include or exclude specific possibilities in its deliberations.

PUBLICATION AND ORGANISATION OF THE OSM KNOWLEDGE BASE

The development of an Oxford System of Medicine could not be treated as a very large conventional software engineering project, like a banking or airline booking system say, some examples of which incorporate upwards of a million lines of computer code. The complexity and cost of creating and maintaining a conventional system which covered enough medicine to be useful to a GP would make the OSM quite impractical. A fundamental requirement of the design, therefore, was that development should take place under the direct editorship of authoritative medical professionals, employing adapted forms of established editorial methods.

The most obvious approach would be to pursue an analogy between the Oxford System of Medicine and a multi-author textbook, such as the two-volume *Oxford Textbook of Medicine* (*OTM*) published by the Oxford University Press. Chapters in this general medical reference work are prepared by individual specialists, under loose editorial guidance. By analogy in the electronic version we might imagine developing a number of loosely related 'specialist' systems, each comparable to a chapter in the book. One specialist would deal with terminal care; others with prescribing in the elderly and gastrointestinal diseases, and so forth. Each system would be largely independent, though presumably with some overall standards concerning the user interface and general approach.

This method soon reveals itself to be inappropriate because it fails to address the need to build and maintain to a high, consistent standard a structure of the size and scope of an OSM. It would permit each expert system to embody different assumptions and approaches to medicine. The knowledge required in different areas could overlap, yet the knowledge organisation used in one module might be incompatible with that in another, leading to unpredictable (and potentially undetectable) gaps and interactions in the knowledge base. Development would be costly, performance poor and different medical areas inconsistent in their operation and facilities. Of course these problems are not new; multi-author books have them too, but unlike computer technology book technology does not demand consistency.

We therefore adopted a different approach which was intended to promote a consistent structure across medical subfields, rather than self-contained specialist systems. The knowledge in the prototype design is organised as sets of modules arranged in layers as illustrated in Figure 13.6. Each module contains information about a topic, written and stored in the computer in a notation that we call 'pseudo-English'.[7] The outermost layer contains sets of medical facts about particular patients, drugs, diseases, etc.

problems of John Smith include gout
side-effects of narcotics include constipation
positive signs of peptic ulcer include epigastric tenderness

The adjoining layer of modules contains information relating topics to each other. A straightforward example is the 'drug hierarchy'. Different classes of drugs, described in publications such as the *British National Formulary*, are represented in the OSM by facts like these:

kinds of drugs include cardiovascular drugs
kinds of cardiovascular drugs include diuretics
kinds of drugs include gastrointestinal drugs

Figure 13.6:

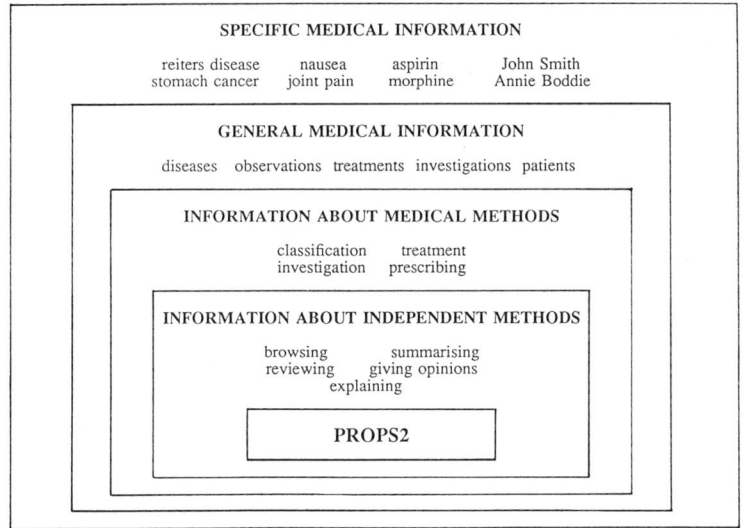

kinds of gastrointestinal drugs include ulcer healing drugs
instances of ulcer healing drugs include cimetidine, . . ., etc.

The next layer is rather different because the modules embody knowledge about how to make medical decisions — diagnosis, treatment, etc. Consequently, as well as facts, they contain 'if . . . then . . .' rules, which specify the steps required to make particular classes of decision. The following example illustrates how we might write an 'if . . . then . . .' rule about making a treatment decision:

if treatment of Problem is required
then find out about any specific form of Problem
and find out about any specific causes of Problem
and find out about any indicants of possible treatments
and find out about any contraindicants of possible treatments
and summarise possible treatments

This is a simplified composite of a number of actual OSM rules, illustrating a number of points. First, although rules like this are equivalent to computer programs they are more easily understood because of the pseudo-English form. Second, this and other treatment rules are 'generalised' to cover all treatment decisions. The capitalised word Problem is a 'logical variable' which could refer to joint pain, anxiety, weight loss, or any other problem whose treatment requires a decision. A consistent approach to the decision irrespective of the details of the problem results.

The final layer of the knowledge base illustrated in Figure 13.6 is like the last in that it contains 'if . . . then . . .' rules, except that these are not specifically medical. They describe how to collect and present information, how to formulate explanations and so forth.

There are several ways in which this modular, layered organisation could support the development, maintenance and electronic publication of medical knowledge on a large scale.

(1) Information about medical topics and decision making methods is in pseudo-English, so is relatively intelligible to editors with more knowledge of medicine than of computer systems.*

(2) The great bulk of the medical knowledge in the system (perhaps a million or so facts in a first edition) is represented as a data base, not as a program. The programs required (generalised medical and domain-independent methods) are small in comparison, perhaps 200–300 rules. Data base maintenance is well established and parts of the process could be automated, whereas maintaining programs is far more difficult.

(3) A clear organisation of the information results from the modularity, making the editorial process simpler.

(4) Representing medical decision-making as a generalised, intelligible procedure allows critical analysis by professionals inside and outside the design time.

A PRINCIPLED APPROACH TO DECISION SUPPORT

Knowledge-based systems emphasise the role of qualitative reasoning in formulating their decisions. The OSM is no exception.

---

* Although the 'pseudo-English' form gives the appearance of being a natural language this is rather deceptive, in that it is still a programming language with a very specific syntax. The question of how far medical authorship can be divorced from a deeper knowledge of the working of the system remains.

However, the decision-making mechanisms of most medical expert systems (most famously in MYCIN, Casnet and Internist) have also made use of quantitative methods for calculating disease probabilities, the expected value of treatments and so on. Although combining quantitative methods with qualitative logical techniques has not been excluded from a future Oxford System of Medicine, no particular emphasis has been placed on this in the prototype.

There are a number of reasons for this apparent omission. Firstly, the available techniques for combining logic and probability are, in our view, *ad hoc* and not based on sound, well-understood principles.[9] Secondly, effective use of mathematical methods depends on the availability of well-estimated statistics, covering the incidence of symptoms and disease, the reliability and value of investigations and so on. These statistics are only available in a small proportion of the areas which concern the general practitioner. Thirdly, we place great value on the intelligibility of the OSM to the medical profession, whereas mathematics may detract from this and turn the 'support' system into a mysterious black box. Quantitative methods offer more precisely calculated decisions, but many practitioners are not convinced that increased precision brings enough advantages to risk losing intelligibility.

One of the great strengths of mathematical decision-making, however, is that its principles are well understood, while those that underlie knowledge-based systems are relatively novel. We must therefore accept a responsibility to develop a framework for decision support in the OSM whose principles are as well motivated as the classical mathematical methods, or are at least equally well described. Satisfying this requirement is currently a major focus of our continuing work on the OSM; we can give a provisional outline here, though a detailed presentation must await a more comprehensive technical paper.

In essence we are trying to state the body of principle — the knowledge — that underlies various forms of medical decision in a form that is available to, and can be used by, a computer. This means that the decision-making knowledge must be expressed in the form of individual 'if . . . then . . .' rules, while treatment decisions, diagnostic decisions etc. are specified by sets of rules in the OSM prototype. These are general in the sense that they are independent of the problem which is being considered. In fact we believe that an even more general procedure may underlie all of the decisions which the OSM can support.

This can be viewed as a choice procedure. Suppose the OSM is required to assist in selecting a treatment for a patient with nausea. Given only this information about the patient some possible causes of the nausea will be apparent (i.e. from facts like 'possible causes of nausea include biliary disease') and some obvious possible treatments ('treatments of nausea include antiemetics'). As more information about this kind of nausea is obtained (e.g. acute or periodic) the set of possible causes changes, and consequently the set of possible treatments may increase or decrease.

For each possible choice of treatment there may be specific indications or contraindications (e.g. the knowledge base contains facts of the form 'contraindications of antiemetics include pregnancy'). Those that are confirmed by the GP represent 'pros' and 'cons' of the possible treatments.

Pros and cons refer to individual choices; interactions between choices must be taken into account as well. For example antiemetics may be indicated, but a more specific indication for metoclopramide may also be present. The decision procedure should recognise that one may subsume the other ('kinds of antiemetics include metoclopramide') and so disregard the more general one. Many relationships can be exploited to reduce the number of possibilities, including relative cost, acceptability to the patient, and so on.

Sometimes a single preferred choice (or combination of choices) remains. If a recommendation is requested that is the one to be offered. Often, however, more than one possibility will remain and an overall quantitative assessment of desirability will be necessary. The last component of the decision procedure is a mechanism for combining the pros and cons in order to make a choice.*

So to summarise the choice procedure:

(1) generate the possible choices (e.g. diagnoses, investigations, treatments);
(2) identify the pros and cons of each choice;
(3) consider possible interactions between the choices;
(4) establish the balance of preference when a single choice must be made.

---

* As remarked it may in future be shown to be desirable and possible to calculate the relative preference for the decision options more precisely. Thus we might calculate the probability of each diagnosis precisely, or the expected information yield of a test or the expected utility of a treatment. Our scheme simply adds up the pros and cons, but if mathematical weights could be validly attached to the pros and cons then more precise calculations could be made without changing the overall logical framework.

SUMMARY AND CAVEATS

In this chapter we have given an introduction to our concept and design of the Oxford System of Medicine. The prototype system which was demonstrated in September 1986 was the result of six months of experimentation aimed at establishing whether a 'publication' like the OSM can realistically be regarded as ripe for development, or whether it is still a goal requiring further research. The prototype contains some 3,000 facts stored in an intelligible and, we believe, maintainable pseudo-English form. These lay down an overall organisation for the medical knowledge base and cover, in some detail, the information required to prescribe about 40 drugs, and the knowledge required for superficial diagnoses, investigation and treatment of joint pain, nausea, breathlessness and other aspects of terminal care. The system can assist with gathering information for these decisions, offer an opinion if required, and account for its conclusions.

We have tried to provide an interface that is both easy to understand and operate, leaving control of what information to provide, and when to provide it, in the user's hands. Ultimately, responsibility and authority for patient management remain with the doctor, and we have tried to avoid deliberately or inadvertently imposing any other regime. A difficulty, however, is that considerable investment is required to find out whether one is even on the right lines. Whether our design, or even a much more developed version of it, is compatible with the complexity, brevity and unpredictability of a consultation will only be certain when it is tried in practice. Evaluation of the effect on patient care will naturally be required; although clinical audit is well established there is relatively little experience in assessing this type of system in general practice.

Our knowledge base of 3000 facts is quite substantial by present standards of the field, but represents only a fragment of a first edition OSM — perhaps a million facts would be needed — though within a few years small computer technology will probably be able to support a system on this scale. The editorial task of expanding the system will be very great, however, and although the separation of factual material from programs promises simplified development and maintenance no-one has yet built a decision support system on the scale of the OSM. The size of the effort required, and the problems of 'scaling up', are to all intents and purposes unknown.

The idea that a generalised method for medical decision-making based on qualitative logic can be developed is a natural, though controversial, consequence of the separation of factual medical knowledge from decision-making principles and user interaction. Medicine tends to be organised and taught around experience, not principles of decision-making. Many will doubt our suggestion that methods for diagnosis, investigation, treatment, etc., can be separated from the details of what you are diagnosing, investigating or treating. If they are correct, and specific medical fields require individual problem-solving techniques, this will have serious implications for the viability of the OSM. The whole knowledge base would require painstaking maintenance by people with programming skills, as well as medical editors, and the development of an OSM would almost certainly be impractical. Although our experience is too limited to draw a firm conclusion we at least are optimistic that medical knowledge can be articulated within a generalised logical framework.

AFTERWORD

The aim of our study was not to produce a practical system, but to ask whether an Oxford system of Medicine is possible and, if so, to demonstrate one realisation of the concept. Although many questions remain the study has led us to the conclusion that an OSM is technically feasible and it, or systems like it, could be successfully built.

The project is continuing with the establishment of an editorial board by the ICRF and OUP. Current research is focused on the three areas of user interface, knowledge base organisation and decision-making techniques discussed above. We hope that this work, in conjunction with developments in electronic publishing at Oxford University Press, will lead to the development of the OSM as a clinically viable tool within the next few years.

ACKNOWLEDGEMENTS

We wish to thank Saki Hajnal for the design and implementation of the window-based interface, and for her critical and constructive comments; also Tim Duncan for much of the work on Props 2.

REFERENCES

1. Pritchard, P. (1985) *The Oxford System of Medicine: report on a feasibility study*. Oxford University Press, Oxford
2. Fox, J., Barber, D. and Bardhan, K.D. (1979) Effects of on-line symptom-processing on history-taking and diagnosis — a simulation study. *International Journal of Biomedical Computing*, *10*, 151–63
3. Fitter, M.J. and Cruickshank, P.J. (1983) Doctors using computers: a case study. In: Sime, M.E. and Coombes, M.J. (eds), *Designing for Human Computer Communication*. Academic Press, London.
4. Barber, D. and Fox, J. (1981) FIRST-AID: A design philosophy and a program for on-line symptom processing. *International Journal of Biomedical Computing*, *12*, 249–65
5. Fox, J. and Rector, A. (1982) Expert systems for primary medical care? *Automedica*, *4*, 123–30
6. Fox, J. and Frost, D. (1985) *Artificial intelligence in primary care*. International Conference on Artificial Intelligence in Medicine, Pavia, Italy. North-Holland, Amsterdam
7. Frost, D., Fox, J., Duncan, T.D. and Preston, J. (1986) *Knowledge engineering through knowledge programming: the Props 2 package*. Imperial Cancer Research Fund, London
8. Buchanan, B.G. and Shortliffe, E.H. (1984) *Rule-based expert systems: the MYCIN experiments of the Stanford Heuristic Programming Project*. Addison Wesley, Reading, Mass.
9. Fox, J. (1986) Knowledge, decision making and uncertainty. In: Gale, W. (ed.), *Artificial Intelligence and Statistics*, Addison Wesley, Reading, Mass.

14

Electronic Technology and Practice Management

Mike Pringle

INTRODUCTION

General practice is at a crossroads and, as never before, the cherished independent contractor status of general practitioners is being examined. We are confronted by the onslaught of computers but we are unsure how to use them effectively. We have pressure on us to change, and particularly to demonstrate and improve our quality of care, but we have little concept of the management of change.

In this chapter I review the current status of practice management and outline the strategies for change that we should all consider. Since information is at the centre of the web of practice management I explore the depths of information that now face modern general practice and the implications of increased information through modern technology. The pressure for information recording in hospitals is already strong[1] and general practitioners have shown themselves willing to be involved in some information collection.[2]

My belief in the need to have a highly skilled practice manager (be it the person with that job title now or a doctor) in each practice to control both information and the changes that it provokes will become apparent. Technology offers us the prospect of controlling our resources and improving our care, and services to our patients. This challenge will be the major task for general practice for the remainder of this century.

THE CHANGING FACE OF MANAGEMENT

In the past 20 years practice managers have changed from curiosity to commonplace. They evolved from the 'senior receptionist' and 'practice book-keepers' roles and now occupy the queen-bee status in practices. Their evolution is a reflection of the increasing complexity of the administration of general practice, not only in the rules and regulations of the general practitioner's contract with the state but also in the areas of wages and salaries, employment law, liability and consumerism. Of these, the last has unique implications in practice management and for practice managers.

Consumerist pressure has, until now, come from the consumers themselves. Patients expect the practice staff to be courteous and efficient. They expect appointments to be available and waiting times to be reasonable. They expect a decent, well-maintained surgery environment. Especially they expect service — repeat prescriptions available quickly and correctly, with reminders when their medication needs reviewing or when preventive care items are due. They expect information to be available on medical and social services matters and for the surgery to respond quickly to their needs for certificates, insurance reports and work medicals. This is all in addition to their primary expectation that their doctors be medically competent, available and skilled in interpersonal relationship and counselling.

One way in which this consumerism has been expressed and controlled is through patient participation groups (PPGs)[3-5] or through practice newsletters.[6] Although the failure rate for PPGs may be high[7] they do offer a rare opportunity in a profession for a dialogue between the consumer and the professional. General practice is unusual since the customer who pays the bill (the NHS) is not directly the consumer (the patient) and medicine has therefore the least financial reason of any profession to respond to consumerism.

It can be argued that many improvements in general practice in recent decades are due to this consumerist pressure reflecting our close relationship with our patients, and the very clear responsibility implicit in the 'registered patient' contract. But it is the nebulous nature of this form of pressure that directly results in the variable standards of care and services that general practice offers. This has led to an increasing profile for the second form of consumerism — from the paying customer.[8] Since the General Practice Charter the Government has had the right by contract to expect an adequate standard of medical care from its independent contractors and has rewarded certain behaviours (item-of-service payments). However, it is now taking an increasing interest in enforcing standards of care, even if its Good Practice Allowance has been dropped.

This particular consumerism will require all the skills of practice management. If patient care is adequate then a practice will need to demonstrate that fact. If targets are set the practice will need to show its progress towards them. It is this dual consumerist demand, from the patient and the NHS, that will place the greatest strain on practice management in the next decade.

It must therefore be asked whether practice managers or practices themselves possess the skills and the information to adapt to these challenges. The answer would appear to be negative. Some practice managers and doctors excel at personnel management. But British general practices are notably poor at information management, and in particular lack the ability to manage change.

This chapter is based on the assumption that until now change has occurred by haphazard doctor-based decision-making, usually with inadequate information. The pressures building up on the discipline of general practice will require the next step forward in our professionalisation. We will need access to high-quality information about our own and our neighbouring practices, and high-quality skills in the management of change. I will deal with these two areas, trying to show how the practice manager is the best-placed person to adopt the control role, and how the introduction of modern technology will make the control of information possible.

MANAGING CHANGE: THE PROCESS

Because of the way they have evolved, practice managers are primarily administrators. Decisions are taken by the doctors, often after consultation with staff, especially the practice manager, and sometimes patients, and are often passed on for implementation. This hierarchical decision-making structure suits the doctors when they are taking decisions which they find easy, and for which the consequences appear clear. Decisions on upgrading the premises are taken alongside the design of the letterhead.

Some decisions, however, appear more complex, such as whether to buy a computer or appoint more staff. At these times the forces in decision-making are reduced to prejudiced reactions, leading to one of two results: the *status quo* is preserved or a poorly researched 'pot-luck' decision is taken. As the finances of the doctors begin to relate directly to the performance of the practice, these two options will increasingly appear inadequate.

Although it is possible that in some practices at least one doctor will assimilate and apply more functional management techniques, it seems likely that this role will increasingly be taken by the practice manager. This is not to assert that the decisions will be taken away from the doctors — only that their decisions will be placed by the manager in the correct context. The information for decision-taking will be established and presented in a comprehensible fashion. The results will be monitored and fed back to the doctors.

If the practice manager is to become this facilitating force — a true 'manager' — then he or she will need to understand and use methods for achieving change. Change can be managed through mandates (contracts, consents, supports) or it can be non-mandated (if either an issue is small or the manager is sufficiently powerful).

There is a limited but positive scope for a manager to effect non-mandated change in general practice. By leading by example in such areas as time-keeping, alertness, compassion and courtesy the attitudes of all the staff, including the doctors, can be influenced. Persuasion can certainly be part of the manager's armoury, but only if it leads to a mandate; there is little benefit in persuading colleagues to allow change if they will obstruct it whenever possible. It is difficult to see how dictatorial management can work except for the most insignificant of decisions — if a practice manager, staff member, doctor or patient is in a position to dictate substantial change then this must have unhealthy consequences for the dynamics of the practice.

The most effective and efficient change will occur through mandates, and a good practice manager should be skilled at creating, defining and maintaining them. These mandates may be expressed through consensus, which would certainly be vital for a very important decision such as whether to move premises. Delegation to subgroups (e.g. the running of the appointments system to the practice manager, one doctor and the senior receptionist) or to individuals (e.g. to the secretary to implement a referral rates monitoring system) is normal and practical, but ultimately depends on the agreement of the whole group.

Management in this sense therefore involves selling ideas and winning people over to experimentation with change. The most effective way of achieving this is by sharing the ownership of ideas with others, but explanation and persuasion are equally acceptable. These are skills that a practice manager requires, but to implement such strategies one needs a mandate from the practice, and especially the doctors, to be this driving force for change.

A manager therefore requires familiarity with the process of

Table 14.1: The steps in managing change and the information required

Definition of problem(s)	Opinions on the problem
Definition of the current position	Past trends Current status Comparative data
Setting targets	Comparative data Past trends
Decide possible strategies	Current resources Available resources Competition for resources Efficiency of application of resources
Intervene	Measurement of progress
Assessment	Measurement of progress Information on other problems Information on resources
Restate targets and strategies, and re-intervene	Measurement of progress Information on other problems Information on resources

change (see Table 14.1). It is for any member of the practice (doctors, staff or patients) to state immediate problems, and it is up to the practice to delegate the task of measuring the current position to a subgroup or individual. Targets are usually set by consensus, but the practice manager is in a pre-eminent place to advise the practice on methodological issues involved and possible strategies, as well as assessing progress and leading re-evaluation. Just who is involved in implementing change depends on who is given the mandate, but the manager is the obvious person to create, define, refine and maintain that mandate.

The power to assume this role will come to practice managers from two sources: the doctors will welcome help with the complex changes that lie ahead, and the managers themselves will assume the power through their acquisition of information. If 'knowledge itself is power'[9] then the same can be said, in modern times, for information.

Practice managers do not yet, however, have information readily available to manage change. They cannot readily define the current position and measure progress. They have no trends on which to superimpose goals, and no continuing information with which to motivate the implementers of change. The most radical prospect that modern technology offers a practice is information, and the practice manager must learn how to use that information to implement change.

MANAGING CHANGE: THE INFORMATION

The increase in complexity of decision-making in general practice that I anticipate in the next decade derives from the demands that will be made on the information systems in the practice, the community and the nation. Practices will increasingly find themselves consulting disparate sources to meet the new demands, and practice development will require a level of planning and supervision far above the current norm.

To see how this can be, the crucial role for information in the management process must be examined. Before controlled change (as opposed to accidental or externally imposed change) can occur it must be justified. This requires, above all, an exact definition of the problem. Unless the problem being addressed is, in fact, the real problem being experienced by a doctor, a member of the primary health care team, or a patient, then the process of change is self-evidently futile.

After defining the problem the next task is to determine how significant it is in terms of the practice. This requires the establishment of a baseline and, if possible, retrospective information to establish trends. If the problem is one of interpersonal relationships between two members of staff, this information is established by interview. As often as not, open discussion of the problem will resolve the conflict. However, it may be necessary to define targets (a more harmonious relationship) and strategies (working different shifts for a few weeks). It can be seen that the model which will be applied to factual information applies equally to other fields like personnel management. The skills are transferable even if the strategies are not.

On a more practical level, let us suppose that the practice wishes to increase uptake of childhood immunisation. The crucial importance of correct management of this task only becomes apparent at the stage of assessing progress. If you don't know where you started from, and you don't know where you've been or even where you want to go to, how can you assess whether your new position is an improvement, or if you have succeeded? It would indeed be a rash organisation that committed resources to the concept of improving a service without information to support that decision, yet that is the reality of much decision-taking in general practice today.

Defining the present, and if possible the past, is therefore of basic importance. It serves two purposes: the practice can compare its performance to its self-expectation and to the performance of other practices (usually national or regional figures), and it can set targets for itself to obtain. Target setting is an art: if too low and easily achievable then complacency ensues; it too high despair replaces optimism and enthusiasm wilts. Targets are often best set as graduated steps, the height of each determined only when the previous rung has been achieved.

Once the practice has decided, after consideration of the baseline and its targets, on the strategies to be adopted, then intervention can occur. Supplementary information may be required throughout this process because it implies choices. The practice may decide that its childhood immunisation rate is, after all, quite adequate and it wishes to put its energy into, say, setting up a patient transport scheme.

Equally the practice may wish to consider resources. It may not have any available receptionist time to set up the call-and-recall system or it might fear that this task will divert attention from another important task such as running a well-man's clinic. It may be that two problems have been identified simultaneously, and that the practice wishes to choose between them. To make any of these choices the practice will require information on which it can base rational judgements.

As the intervention proceeds, the practice requires to know both whether it is being effective and, if it is, how near to the target the action is taking the practice. This requires repetitive monitoring. Not only do such figures allow evaluation of effectiveness but, like a dieter checking his weight, it maintains motivation.

When the practice decides to assess its progress it can see the effect over a period of time. This will show the effect of early enthusiasm, a possible slowing of progress with time, perhaps a further rise as feedback is used to re-motivate. This will allow the practice to set new targets and define new strategies which can be tried. Only high-quality information can allow the practice to evaluate the outcome of its actions in this way.

It might be supposed that only such obvious areas as immunisation rates lend themselves to this information-based approach. However, a consideration of some of the main areas of concern in primary care today shows that this is not the case. Availability and accessibility can be readily monitored by the practice receptionists; the management of chronic disease can be measured in terms of compliance; number of consultations, frequency of examination or investigation and level of control; the level of uptake to preventive care can be quantified; screening rates can be measured; and cost efficiency can be shown through referral rates, investigation rates, prescribing costs, staff costs and equipment expenditure.

To have repetitive accurate information on all these areas is beyond the capacity of the average general practice today. However, modern technology is already offering us some of this information and soon all of it will be there for practices to exploit or ignore. Our challenge is to take this information, develop the management system to apply it and thereby to improve the quality of care we give our communities.

INFORMATION AND ITS SOURCES

Information for practice management, and in particular the management of change, can come from many sources. The appointments book itself yields a wealth of information, both retrospective (seasonal workloads, consultations per patient per year, etc.) and prospective (availability, patient appointment preferences, etc.). The visit book will define visiting patterns and the practice registers will provide data on prevention, repeat prescribing, special need age groups and so on.

Hospitals may offer feedback on referral and investigation rates and may eventually be able to quantify the cost-effectiveness of individual doctors in the use of hospital-based resources. At present they can help a doctor plan his care of individual cases by revealing outpatient waiting times, admission waiting lists and bed occupancy.

Outside bodies can give analyses of performance, such as the prescribing cost of information from the Prescription Pricing Authority. The local authority knows social deprivation indices for the electoral wards covered by the practice, and national data banks hold prescribing and disease information.

It is apparent that a practice may have to trawl wide to have at its disposal the quantity and quality of information that it needs. This analysis of the types of information available now, or which will become available as new technology spreads, is not exhaustive but illustrative, and it will be seen that much can be generated 'in-house'.

Patient-related information

Numbers, ages, sexes and locations

Many practices have this information from either a manual card index age–sex register or a practice computer. Even though crude, information at this level can help a practice to plan well women's clinics, well men's clinics, baby clinics and geriatric screening, should it so wish. It can also help the practice or its PPG to plan transport systems for bringing patients to the surgery, based on the locations of such groups as the elderly or mothers with children.

As the years pass this information can help a practice to see past trends and predict, and anticipate, future ones. Planning for (or justifying) a new partner, closing a branch surgery, or staffing requirements are all influenced by such trends. Such information should be available to a practice which is planning an extension to its premises, or even designing a new building — without such data how can the pitfalls or under- or over-provision be avoided?

Preventive status

Many practices run call-and-recall systems which can inform the manager concerning the number, for example, of cervical smears taken. Some go further and can measure the number of women currently actively smeared, the number who have declined and the number for whom it is inappropriate (having had a hysterectomy, etc.). However, to elicit this information is laborious and the accuracy is seldom high.

Fewer practices can attempt to routinely supply this information for immunisations, blood pressure readings and urine tests. Even many practices with computers find that their programs do not routinely offer analysis of the preventive level in the practice. Yet practices set up call-and-recall systems, preventive item opportunistic reminders or start local health education campaigns with no evidence on the size of the problem and no attempt to measure the effectiveness of their intervention. It appears that the objective is to be seen to be acting, rather than having an effect — to be pleasing the consumer not the customer.

Only when practices have information on the current status and past trends, preferably with local and national figures for comparison, can an efficient preventive care programme be sustained. The evolving pattern will show how effective the chosen strategy is, and will help to motivate the doctors and staff to continue their interest in the programme.

Morbidity

Morbidity is the bread-and-butter of general practice, and it is difficult at first to see how measuring it can be of more than ephemeral interest. But there are two good reasons for doing so. Firstly it is not possible to propose, or to argue against, a special clinic (diabetic mini-clinic, nurses' hypertension clinic or a well men's clinic) without knowing the incidence of diabetes, hypertension or ischaemic heart disease in the practice.

It is not until such information is compared to regional and national figures that local idiosyncrasies can be identified. For example, I have become aware that my practice has a higher incidence of multiple sclerosis and urinary tract cancer than would be normally expected. Only last year did the doctors of South Derbyshire discover they were in the national black spot for myocardial infarction — and it took the District Health Authority to demonstrate it.

The second reason for morbidity recording relates to quality of care. Many general practitioners are already setting out protocols for their management of diseases. In the case of diabetes this might include the aim of examining the fundi and feeling foot pulses every year, and taking blood for glycosylated haemoglobin and blood sugar every six months. If such protocols are to be effective they must be monitored, requiring easy, accurate identification of the relevant disease group and the auditing of their clinical records.

Mortality information

An increase in local mortality, in one disease or overall, can have such complicated causes as to be of limited value. However, there is a good case to be made for a practice to examine the notes of all sudden deaths, and deaths from myocardial infarction or cerebrovascular accident. This can help highlight failures to record blood pressure or follow up high readings, family histories of ischaemic heart disease that were ignored or smokers that were not counselled. A mortality register can help to stimulate and resource such meetings.

Prescribing information

The Prescription Pricing Authority (PPA) has for some years offered feedback to general practitioners on their prescribing costs. These analyses are for one month only, relate to the doctor whose name appears on the prescription (not always the prescriber, by any means) and give a limited 'snapshot' on the number of items prescribed, the cost per item and the cost per registered patient.

While this initiative can be applauded it illustrates how a little information can whet the appetite for more. A high-cost prescriber is entitled to feel perplexed. This information informs but it does not explain. There is no clue as to what drugs are being over-prescribed and whether, indeed, this problem is in all drug groups. It is all too easy to dismiss such information as 'atypical' or 'irrelevant'.

Therefore the PPA now supplies on request to prescribing doctors a very detailed computer analysis of a practice's prescribing, allowing the problem areas to be clearly identified and discussed. What effect this has on subsequent prescribing is as yet uncertain, but there is evidence that such information can be beneficial in the short term.[10,11]

Practices can generate information most easily from repeat prescriptions, especially if these are computer-generated. From such analyses a practice can move towards a practice formulary and monitor progress. It can also adopt policies concerning, say, the repeat prescribing of psychotropics.

Appointments and availability

The best care in the world is futile if a patient cannot be seen, and the availability of urgent appointments and routine appointments with individual doctors can be monitored on a day-to-day, week-to-week basis. It may become apparent that one doctor is more unavailable than the others in a practice, and this would be best discussed within the partnership before problems occur. It might be that non-surgery workloads need adjusting or the partner needs to look at the number of follow-up appointments he requests patients to make.

The length of time a patient waits in the surgery is an old chestnut, but it is often a cause of much patient disquiet. Ways have been described to analyse the waiting times and redesign the appointments booking interval to closely match consultation length, giving a minimum wait both for doctors and patients.[12] To do this requires information on consulting rates, and patient and doctor waiting times.

Delivery of health care information

Encounter information

By measuring both the number of doctor–patient encounters and their location, a practice manager can build up a perception of changing demand[13] and of individual and practice workloads. When published, such figures[14] can result in misinterpretation, but they can be helpful in identifying, say, the partner most available to take on a new commitment such as an old persons' home.

Investigations

Most pathology laboratories are computerised, and it would not require extensive alterations to their programs for all local doctors to be given details of their usage broken down by type of investigation requested, and comparative values for their partners, other local practices and regional or national averages. Radiography departments are, by and large, not yet computerised, but there is the scope for similar analyses.

It may be that individual practices may choose to do their own information gathering in such areas if either the range or the depth of hospital-generated recording were too limited. It might, for example, not just want to look at sheer numbers but to analyse by the intention (to exclude, to confirm, to monitor, etc.) and whether the result was normal or abnormal, expected or unexpected. In this case a conventional one-off audit could be done, but if continuous information were required then a computer would be invaluable.

Referrals, admissions and discharges

Hospital computers are already being applied to bed occupancy and the assessment of relative cost efficiency between teams. Although they do not routinely supply this information in digestible form to primary care, the capacity to do so exists. If a practice is to understand the movements of its patients and assess, for example, the implications of a policy for a nurse to visit every postoperative discharge, then it must have this information from all the hospitals for each doctor. But this information may best be recorded within the practice. Whether a computer is needed to record this information depends largely on the extent of the recording and the uses the practice visualises for it. A simple paper register of referrals and admissions with principal diagnosis kept over, say, three months, may suffice to discern trends. However, most practices will start to expect these data on a regular basis once they have started to collect them.

Practice turnover

If a practice is to know who it serves it must have a tool for defining that population. Age–sex registers, computerised or manual, serve this purpose. The turnover within such a register can, however, be more difficult to measure directly, and this is usually done by counting the number of records requested back by, and received from, the Family Practitioner Committee (FPC). The FPC can, using their computers, give practices the same figures.

While it would hardly justify a computer on its own, a practice computerised age–sex register should be giving information on turnover, not just registration totals. Unfortunately most do not do this. The information could be used for predicting workload bulges (especially in practices with high student numbers) and for planning practice size. Since a small change in the registration rate in high-turnover practices can have a dramatic effect on practice population numbers, the size of turnover, and its causes, need to be known and observed.

Community support

Two trends are discernible in recent decades. The community in human terms is becoming less caring in its support of the elderly and the chronic sick, delegating more and more of the responsibility to the 'Social Services'. Caring is becoming professionalised. However, the second and equally worrying trend is for society (including the medical community) to expect a single person (usually a relative) to take on the role of carer with little support or appreciation.

If a practice is to become the interface between the needs of the patients and the resources of the state, and between the inadequacies of the state and the pressure on carers, then it will require both commitment and information. It will need to know what is available and where the needs are greatest. It may be that a manual register of those patients living alone, those dependent on a career, those receiving mobility or attendance allowance and those identified (e.g. through geriatric screening) as being at risk can be constructed. The social performance index for each patient could be measured and recorded.[15]

The more the scope for such a register is realised, the more apparently it should be linked to other indices such as morbidity and admissions, to location and repeat prescribing, to number of encounters and investigation rates. This concept of record linkage is not new,[16,17] but it can become a reality through the imaginative use of computers within the practice environment.

Cost-efficiency information

Increasingly the DHSS is going to expect primary care to demonstrate value for money. There is, however, a fundamental issue to be confronted. Just measuring process is inadequate unless the quality of decisions is taken into account. If two doctors have identical referral rates one might be referring some patients unnecessarily while not referring others who need it. If one doctor refers more than the average it might be because he is screening more patients and detecting more illness in its early stages, or it might be because he recognises his areas of ignorance and uses the referral to save his patient from himself. It is difficult to criticise such insight, even if it might be a reason for educational intervention.

Practices might, however, wish to compare efficiency using referral rates, equipment costs and staffing levels to increase awareness of areas of concern, and highlighting differences. While such comparisons cannot be judgemental, since each practice is influenced by so many internal and external factors, they can be used to increase insight into resource and cost implications.

Community information

Primary care is, possibly, unique in that it consists of small businesses with sizeable turnover and staffing, but with little information on the current and future demand for its services. Many practices may find an increased awareness of community dynamics would help in the planning of services and in making the case for resources; for example expansion of the primary health care team. The census asks for information on social conditions including housing, income and car ownership. For each electoral ward a deprivation profile is constructed, and this is available to the local authority and the District Health Authority, and to general practices on request.

Using patient addresses (and especially the postcode) the relative social status of a practice can be drawn up in such terms that a forceful case can be made for resource allocation. Allied to this, information on community needs (single elderly, single-patient families) and idiosyncratic morbidity/mortality trends can be used. The rate of provision of nursing home places, sheltered accommodation and special housing for the handicapped and elderly can be calculated, and practice planning adjusted accordingly.

One practical method of using modern technology to aid the social care of the community is through advice on welfare benefits.[18,19] The benefits system is notoriously complex, but Jarman has created a program to help patients to assess their entitlement and to compare the outcomes from various claim strategies.

The hospital community interface provides another valuable source of information. Bed occupancy (especially in general practice maternity wings), waiting times for outpatient appointment and admission, and the availability of hospital transport can all help both doctor and patient choose the most appropriate routes for secondary referral. This information is often already known, but is not very available. However, in time it should be accessible through either a local network system or the practice computer's data base. Equally the practitioner will need to know the bed state and availability in the local nursing homes, old persons' homes and sheltered accommodation for short- and long-term admissions, and this information could be available through a local information network.

National and local data bases

Already Prestel offers doctors drug interaction, clinical and pathology information. Patients have their own data bases on common diseases to consult. Patients will have increasing access to major sources of information which will offer them information that will require interpretation and explanation. The implications for practice management are substantial. If a practice is to respond to patient concerns aroused by reading screens of information then it must be aware of the content of those screens — it must have access to the same data banks.

There are other data banks that can prove invaluable for the practice. Already many doctors use computerised indices of the medical literature to do searches for relevant articles and books. These information tools can also now allow the searcher to read an abstract of the article on the screen to see if it is really the one required. Soon practitioners will have poisons information, drug interaction and choice, and 'textbook' medical information to consult.

Locally, patients will soon expect to be able to check availability of general practice consultations and make appointments through their local network, and practices will expect to book outpatient appointments at the local hospital through a computer connection. If money can be transferred through computers there is no reason why appointments should not be handled. The two biggest blocks are the cost of the technology and the belief of the users. Both these will be surmounted in the next few years.

BRINGING IT ALL TOGETHER

Facts surround us, but usually they are obscured by the activities of daily work. Paper systems are adequate at drawing attention to a few facts, but are not suited to continuous recording. Practice management, either by practice managers or doctors, requires, first and foremost, facts and then the skills to apply management techniques to achieve change. The wealth of information that can be useful to decision-making in general practice is clear, but until now it has been impossible to attempt to have all of it available to the decision-makers. Developments in electronic technology mean that computerised practices will be able to collect information about all aspects of practices' activities — the data being routinely abstracted and brought together for analysis.

The possibility of an integrated patient record with those items of information required for planning clearly linked together to allow flexible and meaningful analysis is clear. The accumulation of this information over time to allow trends to emerge is vital, as is the ability to assess the results of the application of strategies for change. The possibilities inherent in local and national information networks are vast but, as yet, unproven. However, practices need to bear in mind the changes that may occur when planning their services today.

The most radical changes that will accrue from the information revolution will be based on the role of the practice manager. From planning will come the ability to be proactive rather than reactive, to respond to real need rather than imagined need, to demonstrate quality of care rather than aspire to it. The challenge to the independent contractor status of the general practitioner is clear. In this chapter I have attempted to show how, with the aid of developing technology, that challenge can be met and primary care can become a force for change into the twenty-first century.

REFERENCES

1. Korner, E. (1983) (Chairman) *Report of steering group on Health Services Information*. DHSS, London
2. Fraser, R.C. and Gosling, J.T.L. (1985) Information systems for general practitioners for quality assessment. *British Medical Journal, 291*, 1473–6
3. Pritchard, P. (ed.) (1981) *Patient participation in general practice*. Occasional Paper 17. Royal College of General Practitioners, London
4. Hutton, A. and Robins, S. (1985) What the patient wants from patient participation. *Journal of the Royal College of General Practitioners, 35*, 133–5
5. Petrie, J. (1986) Publicising patient participation groups. *British Medical Journal, 293*, 369–70
6. Practice Participation Association (1986) Practice newsletter: three years experience. *British Medical Journal, 293*, 793–4
7. Mann, R. (1985) Why Patient Participation Groups stop functioning: general practitioner's viewpoint. *British Medical Journal, 290*, 209–11
8. Department of Health and Social Security (1986) *Primary Health Care — An Agenda for Discussion*. HMSO, London
9. Bacon, F. (c. 1598) Religious meditations: Of heresies
10. Harris, C.M., Jarman, B., Woodman, E., White, P. and Fry, J.S. (1984) *Prescribing — a suitable case for treatment*. Occasional Paper 24. Royal College of General Practitioners, London
11. Harris, C.M., Fry, J.S., Jarman, B. and Woodman, E. (1985) Prescribing — a case for prolonged treatment. *Journal of the Royal College of General Practitioners, 35*, 284–7
12. Marshall, E.I. (1986) Waiting for the doctor. *British Medical Journal, 292*, 993–5
13. Fry, J. and Dillone, J.B. (1986) Workload in general practice 1950–85. *Journal of the Royal College of General Practitioners, 36*, 403–4
14. Wilkin, D. and Metcalfe, D.H.M. (1981) List size and patient contact in general medical practice. *British Medical Journal, 289*, 1501–5
15. Williams, E.I. (1986) A model to describe social performance levels in elderly people. *Journal of the Royal College of General Practitioners, 36*, 422–3
16. Acheson, E.D. (ed.) (1986) *Record Linkage in Medicine*. Livingstone, Edinburgh
17. Crombie, D. (1981) Record linkage in automated systems. *Journal of the Royal College of General Practitioners, 31*, 325–6
18. Jarman, B. (1985) Giving advice about welfare benefits in general practice. *British Medical Journal, 290*, 522–4
19. Buckle, J. (1986) Informing patients about attendance and mobility allowances. *British Medical Journal, 293*, 1077–8

15

Health Information for Patients

Neil Carson and Peter MacIsaac

Until recently, computer use in medicine has been limited to those involved in the delivery of health care. However, change in technology and the increasing familiarity that the public have with computers now makes it possible for patients to use computers directly. The technological elements responsible for this change include the availability of inexpensive microcomputer systems which can be simultaneously accessed by a number of people, and the development of systems capable of use by those who possess no specialist computer knowledge.

Through direct contact with the computer, patients will be able to enter information and use the computer as a source of information on health and illness. This chapter will describe some examples of what we can term the patient–computer interface. The first examples chosen will be those that require the presence of an operator such as the doctor, where the patient is an indirect user. The second group of examples described are those where the patient is a direct user and is seated at the terminal.

Indirect use
Patient education
Patient instruction
Drug information
Direct use
Data collection and analysis
Learning from the computer

PATIENT EDUCATION AND INSTRUCTION

In recent years there has been increased emphasis on the doctors' role in illness education, preventive care and health promotion. There is a need to supplement and reinforce the verbal component of the consultation. In response to this need a wide range of patient 'hand-outs' have been developed by medical journals, the pharmaceutical industry and special interest groups such as cancer societies, hospitals and self-help groups. The quality and effectiveness of this *patient educational material* has varied. Some suffer from an information overkill, and others from inappropriate use of technical language. Often they become unavailable as stocks run out.

Using the computer for storage will overcome the problem of storage and access, and will limit consulting room clutter. Material can be altered by simple word processing if required, so that individual doctors can control the information they are supplying. A prototype of such a system has already been developed,[1] and is designed to stand alone or to be linked with the medical record. If so linked the printed material can automatically incorporate the patient's own name in the body of the document, so increasing its educational power.

By using diagrams the video-screen itself can be used to provide the patient with simple graphic descriptions of the nature of the problem during a consultation. An important secondary result of the use of the screen in this way is to encourage the patient's involvement with the computer and thereby to improve patient comfort with the computer equipment in the consulting room. A take home print-out is then provided to reinforce the verbal and visual information provided during the consultation.

An example of such a screen is shown in Figure 15.1. It is designed to assist in the education of a patient suffering oesophageal reflux or 'heartburn'. In addition to the drawing of the stomach (one with and one without an associated hiatus hernia) there is a brief list of important points to remind the doctor to discuss with the patient. Figure 15.2 shows the print-out of such a screen. Doctors may wish to write their own patient education material, in which case we have listed a few guidelines (see Table 15.1).

Patient instructions are very similar to illness education, but may not require the use of the screen in the consulting room. The computer merely acts as a convenient word processor and storage cabinet for instructions such as those issued after head injury, or those describing how a patient should collect specimens of urine or

Figure 15.1: Patient education screen

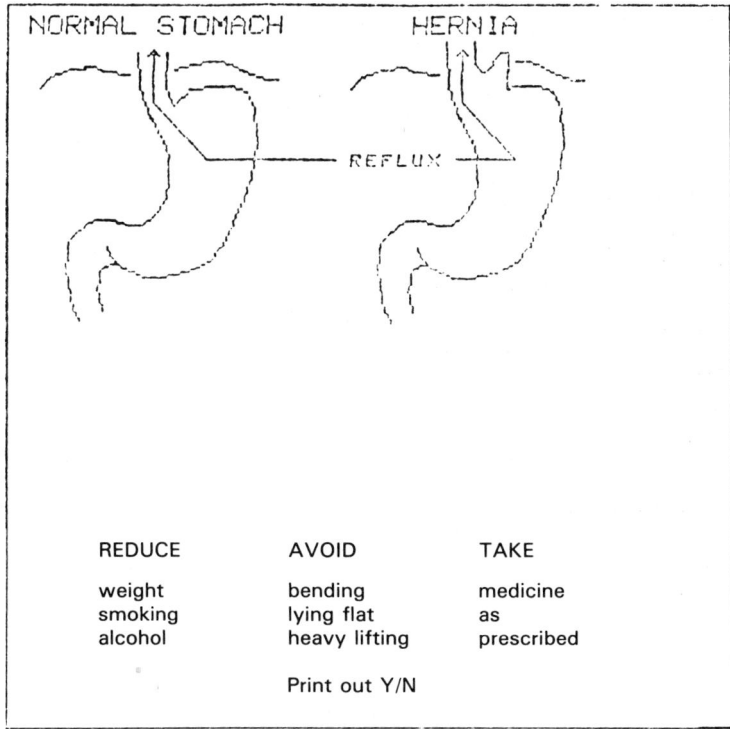

semen for analysis, or listing those precautions to be taken after the application of a plaster cast. By linking these print-outs to the medical record, personalisation and dating of the instructions can be automatically achieved.

The computer system which provides patient education and instructions needs to be rapidly accessible, so that during the consultation the doctor can either proceed through a menu (a classified list of available screens and print-outs) or by direct access through keying in the appropriate descriptive words or a range of equivalents. In our 'heartburn' example described above, this may be accessed through a list (menu) or by keying in a range of alternatives such as 'reflux', 'H.H.', 'oesophagitis' or 'heartburn'.

Figure 15.2: Patient education print-out

Mrs. J. Thompson — 13 Smith Street, Bentleigh.

PATIENT EDUCATION — "HEART BURN"

At times you may have noticed: —

1. A burning chest discomfort
2. Central tenderness below your ribs
3. An acid taste in your mouth

This is caused by the return (or reflux) of strongly acid stomach contents into the throat. Normally this does not happen.
Reflux happens because: —

1. A ring of muscle at the lower end of the oesophagus does not close effectively   OR
2. There is a Hiatus Hernia.

If reflux is prevented you will obtain relief from your discomfort.

To prevent reflux: —

    REDUCE — weight
                — smoking
                — alcohol intake

    AVOID   — bending
                — lying flat in bed. Elevate the bed-head using 2 bricks
                — heavy lifting
                — straining (especially at the toilet)

    TAKE   — medicine as prescribed e.g. antacids

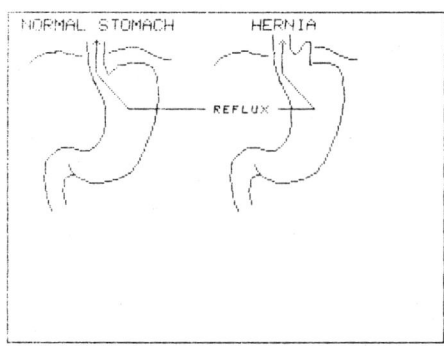

Table 15.1: Some guidelines for preparation of patient information

1. *Be brief*	Limit the amount of information to a single screen and the print-out to a maximum of one page.
2. *Be selective*	Use only the most important information and exclude that which is likely to be rarely required.
3. *Focus on objectives*	The information is designed to educate the patient about the problem and to encourage effective involvement in management. Avoid any other material.
4. *Avoid jargon*	Carefully edit all material to eliminate medical jargon and technical language.

DRUG INFORMATION

The pharmaceutical industry is thriving, with more drugs available than ever before. The future promises further developments including possible antiviral and anticancer agents. With all these benefits comes the problem of increased risk of iatrogenic disease and patient compliance difficulties. It is no longer possible for doctors to keep all this expanding knowledge in their heads, and rapid reference systems are essential. Specific contraindications exist to the use of many drugs, such as beta-blockers in patients with asthma. Care in prescribing is required to avoid side-effects and drug interactions, some of which may be life-threatening. Further, the uncertain risks of drug use in pregnancy, and the possibility of problems occurring in children of lactating mothers, now need to be seriously considered.

A single-screen drug information system has been prepared for the use of doctors in the consulting room while the patient is present.[2,3] The screen has been designed in a standardised format (see examples in Figures 15.3 and 15.4). The problem immediately arises that there are occasions when the single-screen 'rule' does not permit all the information required to be displayed in a readable fashion. In these instances a ' + ' sign appears at the end of a segment of information, which draws attention to the existence of an extra screen of information. This second or 'verbose' screen can be readily accessed and the additional information is displayed (Figure 15.5). Although this information is available as a print-out, and may

Figure 15.3: Drug information screen — framework

identification..

description..

indications..

contraindications..................................

pregnancy-lactation.............................

side-effects..

interactions..

N.H.S.*...

dose - adult...

dose - paediatric..................................

comments...

more information..................................

*N.H.S.(Australia) refers to National Health service details.

Dosages are listed according to N.H.S. requirements.

be useful at times with well-educated patients, generally it will be too technical and will not match the patient's needs and expectations. A simpler and more useful print-out format is shown in Figure 15.6. These hand-outs are designed to be printed when the patient is first prescribed a drug, although they could be re-issued if required at every request for repeat prescriptions. There are a number of difficulties in designing drug information, including those rules listed in Table 15.1. Many side-effects reported are extremely rare and not necessarily proven. There are many drugs where a complete list of all adverse effects is so large it would dissuade any reasonable patient from taking the risk of using that therapy. A balance needs

Figure 15.4: Drug information screen — example for digoxin

id	digoxin lanoxin lanoxin pg
desc	cardiac glycoside
indic	congestive cardiac failure; atrial tachyarrhythmias
contra	current digitalis toxicity, ventricular tachycardia; care in hypokalaemia, smaller doses with impaired renal function
preg-lact	probably safe
side-effects	serious: arrhythmias common: bradycardia, ecg changes, nausea, vomiting, anorexia, diarrhoea, abdominal pain, fatigue, malaise, headache, muscle weakness, neuralgia, drowsiness, blurred and yellow vision +
interact	diuretics, corticosteroids, amphotericin b — hypokalaemia
nhs	tab lanoxin pg 62.5 mcg 100's 2 rpt tab lanoxin 250 mcg 50's 2 rpt elixir 50 mcg/ml 100 ml 2 rpt
dose-adult	125-500 mcg/day in 1 or 2 divided dose
dose-paed	10-20 mcg/kg/day
comments	use extreme caution with rapid oral/in digitalisation
more info	mims annual 1984 p. 88

Figure 15.5: Verbose display

side-effects	serious:	arrhythmias
	common:	bradycardia, ecg changes, nausea, vomiting, anorexia, diarrhoea, abdominal pain, fatigue, malaise, headache, muscle weakness, neuralgia, drowsiness, blurred and yellow vision +
	less common:	
	cvs:	deterioration in c.c.f
	skin:	rash
	gi:	haemorrhage
	general:	gynaecomastia
	haem:	thrombocytopenia, eosinophilia
	cns:	disorientation, confusion, aphasia, delirium, hallucination, convulsion

to be struck between providing excessive or irrelevant information and providing insufficient detail to be of any real value. The examples shown are hopefully ways around this problem. It is the belief of the authors that this type of information should be provided by the prescribing doctor. There are a number of drug information systems used in Australia by pharmacists, and already there is

Figure 15.6: Example of drug information designed for the patient — either as a screen or a print-out

PATIENT DRUG INFORMATION

Patient's name Mr George

ZANTAC
for treatment of peptic ulcers

Brand name: Zantac

Chemical name: ranitidine

What is Zantac?: Zantac reduces the production of acid from the cells in the stomach wall. It is used to treat ulcers, and reflux oesophagitis.

What is the dose? Two tablets a day. After your problem has settled your doctor may direct you to take only one a day.

When and how is it taken? One tablet in the morning and one at night, or two at night. It does not matter whether it is taken before or after meals.

What is the length of treatment? Usually four to six weeks but as advised by your doctor. Do not miss any doses.

Is it safe for children? Yes but an accidental overdose requires prompt action. Ring your doctor or the poisons information centre.

Is it safe during pregnancy and breast feeding? It is not known exactly at this stage if Zantac is safe.

What are the unwanted effects (side effects)? A few patients may develop problems such as headache, nausea, diarrhoea, tiredness and a skin rash.

What about alcohol and other drugs? Apart from upsetting the stomach alcohol is not a problem but antacids can affect Zantac. Discuss this issue of clashing of drugs with your doctor or pharmacist.

What are the special rules to follow?
- continue other anti ulcer advice such as ceasing alcohol and smoking
- report any unusual symptoms to your doctor.

anecdotal evidence suggesting that on occasions inappropriate information has persuaded some patients to stop their medication. The doctor is in a better relationship with the patient to be selective about the information provided.

We have referred to patient education which may be provided directly or indirectly through a health professional. We now look at the direct use of the computer by a patient.

DATA COLLECTION AND ANALYSIS

The futuristic view of a patient being interviewed by a computerised diagnostician is currently far from achievable, given the complexities of medical interviewing and the diagnostic process. However, computers will increasingly be used to question patients in specific and limited areas. In this way patients can provide the routine components of their medical history, or be questioned on lifestyle, prevention, diet and drug use. This information is currently collected in the medical interview or by questionnaire. The direct entry of this information by the patient allows the complex analysis of this information to be immediately available to both doctor and patient.

The check-up

The value of the 'annual medical' or 'check-up' is seriously being questioned. The traditional response to such a request has been a limited medical history followed by a general physical examination and some tests. An alternative approach is the identification of specific health risks that apply to the individual patient. This takes into account factors such as the patient's age, sex, past and family history, occupation, stress and lifestyle. Much of the information collected is of a standard or routine nature, and can be analysed to provide information on health risks and the development of preventive strategies for the individual patient.

A 'Health Risk Appraisal' program has been developed by the Centers for Disease Control, USA, and is currently being modified for use in Australia.[4] This program runs on IBM microcomputers and is designed to collect the relevant data and analyse health risks based on Australian mortality statistics.

Figure 15.7 is a portion of a 'print-out' adapted from this

Figure 15.7: Adapted from the Shepherd Foundation Health Risk Appraisal Printout

HEALTH RISK APPRAISAL

Name: Janet Smith

Actual age: 30 years
Health Age: 36 years
Achievable Health Age: 32 years
Possible improvement   4 years

* Health Age is a measure of how healthy you are compared to others of your sex.

* Achievable Health Age is an estimate of how healthy you could be by making the following changes in your condition or lifestyle.

HEALTH FACTOR	CURRENT	DESIRABLE
EXERCISE	NIL	SEDENTARY EXERCISE PROGRAM
CHOLESTEROL	7.0	BELOW 5.5
BP: DIASTOLIC	100	88
ALCOHOL	24 GLASSES WINE/WEEK	3-6 GLASSES WINE/WEEK
CANCER OF BREAST	NO SELF EXAMINATION	MONTHLY SELF EXAMINATION
CERVICAL SMEAR	NIL	EVERY 2ND YEAR
WEIGHT	85 KG	66 KG.

program. In addition it lists the risk of death from the common causes of mortality for that individual's age and sex.

What you eat

The relationship between diet and many diseases has long been recognised. An assessment of a patient's diet is helpful in the diagnosis and treatment of conditions such as obesity and hypercholesterolaemia. This assessment is made after taking a dietary history followed by an analysis of the composition of the diet. This is a time-consuming and specialised task which is usually performed by dieticians.

A computer program under development by the CSIRO Division of Human Nutrition[5] will provide a computerised self-administered dietary analysis. This program is based on a diet analysis program used in dietary research projects, and collects information on various foods consumed, analyses the component nutrients and provides dietary advice.

Figure 15.8 is an example of one segment of the computerised dietary analysis feedback.[6] The computer print-out also contains an analysis of the average daily intake of important nutrients. Programs such as this will be of use to doctors and other health workers who

Figure 15.8: Computerised dietary analysis feedback

YOUR DIET WAS FOUND TO BE SIGNIFICANTLY HIGHER THAN RECOMMENDED FOR:

- ● PROTEIN — IN YOUR DIET MAJOR SOURCES WERE:
  .... RED MEAT & MEAT PRODUCTS (29%)
  .... DAIRY PRODUCTS (21%)

- ● SUGARS — IN YOUR DIET MAJOR SOURCES WERE:
  .... NON-ALCOHOLIC BEVERAGES (27%)
  .... DAIRY PRODUCTS (15%)
  .... YELLOW/ORANGE FRUIT (14%)
  REFINED SUGARS WERE MAINLY FROM:
  .... NON-ALCOHOLIC BEVERAGES (27%)

- ● TOTAL FAT — IN YOUR DIET MAJOR SOURCES WERE:
  .... DAIRY PRODUCTS (27%)
  .... RED MEAT & MEAT PRODUCTS (18%)

- ● SAT. FATS — IN YOUR DIET MAJOR SOURCES WERE:
  .... DAIRY PRODUCTS (35%)
  .... BUTTER OR MARGARINE (18%)

- ● CHOLESTEROL — IN YOUR DIET MAJOR SOURCES WERE:
  .... RED MEAT & MEAT PRODUCTS (40%)
  .... DAIRY PRODUCTS (18%)

- ● SODIUM (SALT) — IN YOUR DIET MAJOR SOURCES WERE:
  .. SAVOURY DISHES (EG PIZZA, STEW) (28%)
  .... RED MEAT & MEAT PRODUCTS (17%)

YOUR DIET WAS FOUND TO BE SIGNIFICANTLY LOWER THAN RECOMMENDED FOR:

- ● STARCHES — GOOD SOURCES ARE:
  CEREAL PRODUCTS (LOW SALT, UNREFINED)
  STARCHY VEGETABLES (EG POTATO)
  (NOT FRIED)

- ● FIBRE — GOOD SOURCES ARE:
  CEREAL PRODUCTS (LOW SALT, UNREFINED)
  STARCHY VEGETABLES (EG POTATO)
  (NOT FRIED)
  .... LEAFY/ORANGE/RED VEGETABLES

- ● ● ● ● IT HAS BEEN NOTED WITH INTEREST THAT YOUR DIET CONTAINS OVER TEN TIMES THE MINIMUM DAILY REQUIRED OF:
  VITAMIN C
  VITAMIN B1
  VITAMIN B2

need to advise patients on diet but do not have the skills needed for dietary analysis.

LEARNING FROM THE COMPUTER

For many years computers have been used in schools, universities and colleges as teaching aids. The techniques used in computer-assisted learning by students and undergraduates will be applied in future to educate patients about health and illness.

A large proportion of the workload of the modern doctor involves the treatment of chronic or long-term illness. Diseases such as diabetes, hypertension and osteoarthritis have no 'cure', and so both patient and doctor are involved in their long-term management. It is now recognised that in these types of problems the patient himself has a major role to play in the management of his own problem. Factors such as lack of knowledge, unresolved concerns and a failure of commitment to the treatment plan can seriously undermine the effectiveness of medical treatment. Education of patients with chronic illness is an area where computer-assisted learning can play a major role. The advantages of computer education include its suitability for both self-learning and use in groups. Material can be updated and adapted for local use, and can be used over and over again.

Diabetes

The management of patients with insulin-dependent diabetes is an example of a complex management situation. It requires not only the correct use of insulin, but also a degree of understanding by the patient of the physiology of glucose metabolism and the pharmacology of medication.[7] In addition a detailed dietary knowledge, and an understanding of the cause and treatment of diabetic emergencies, is essential. The patient must also possess skills in blood sugar monitoring and injection techniques.

Education is a central component of diabetic management plan, and many diabetic treatment centres have trained educators. Faced with an increasing client load, and restricted financial resources, many educators are turning to the use of computers. A problem with some of the currently available diabetes education programs is that

Figure 15.9: Two screens adapted from Lesson 2 of 'Diabetes Key Facts'

DIABETES KEY FACTS - LESSON 2

Question 1

First off, I need to find out if you know what hypoglycaemia means.

Choose the range of blood glucose levels which you think represents hypoglycaemia.

- A.   below about 3.5 mmol/l
- B.   3.5 - 8 mmol/l
- C.   4 - 10 mmol/l
- D.   anything below 5 mmol/l
- E.   I think I know, but would like it explained anyway

Question 2

Now choose the TWO groups of people in whom hypoglycaemia can occur:

- A.   Those who do not have diabetes
- B.   Those with diabetes treated just with DIET
- C.   Those with diabetes treated with TABLETS
- D.   Those with diabetes treated with INSULIN

---

they do not operate on commonly available personal computers. In some, dedicated and expensive hardware is required. However the situation is changing.

Dr Mathew Cohen, an Australian consultant specialising in diabetes, has developed a computer-based learning program for both insulin-dependent and non-insulin-dependent diabetics. 'Diabetes Key Facts'[8] consists of ten lessons each of 20–30 minutes duration, and operates on the IBM range of microcomputers. It is written using an 'authoring program',[9] which allows educators who are not computer programmers to develop computer based lessons.

Figure 15.9 shows screens adapted from the lesson on hypoglycaemia.

Before answering the questions posed by the program the user is presented with information on blood sugar metabolism. All answers are rewarded with positive feedback. If the answer given is incorrect the user is directed through screens of further information and testing until the essential concepts are grasped. The authoring system used for this lesson provides for several different types of questions such as true/false and free-text entry. Additional features include the use of colour, graphics, sound and animation which increase the impact of the message on the user.

Computer-assisted learning allows the lesson to proceed at a rate suitable to the individual, and this program incorporates the facility to check the level of understanding before proceeding to the next topic. In diabetes education this approach assists the patient to acquire the large volume of factual knowledge required. Preliminary use of this educational program has shown that, while not replacing traditional teaching methods, it provides an effective option for teaching patients about their condition.

In the course of the program 'Diabetes Key Facts' uses a number of educational strategies. The first is question and answer with feedback immediately provided. Based on the response, the program then either branches to provide new information or proceeds to the next item. The second is a 'tutorial' format, where new information is first presented and a 'looping' back facility enables revision. The third strategy is that of simulation, using a real case example such as a hypoglycaemic episode.

'Diabetes Key Facts' is an example of one of the ways in which a computer can be used in patient education. The future will see many similar programs once health educators begin to explore the possibilities of the computer as a teaching aid.

CONCLUSION

Computers in medicine have until now been performing mainly administrative tasks. They will soon be moving from the 'back room' and will be used by health professionals and their patients for education and data collection.

We have described the important role we foresee for the computer in providing educational material both inside and outside the consultation.

The advantages of patient-operated data collection programs include:

1. the time spent by patients waiting to see the doctor can be better utilized;
2. time savings for the doctor and staff in collection and analysis of information;

3. well-designed computer questionnaires can make it easier for patients to provide an accurate reply to sensitive or embarrassing questions;
4. the computer never becomes tired or forgets a question, and any missing or incomplete data can be readily identified.

As with any tool, however, computerised questionnaires and instructions have a number of limitations. Important information may be missed if it is outside the scope of the program and the computer analysis may be open to misinterpretation. Patients must be comfortable with using a computer, and need to be literate. While it is likely that programs such as those described will be used increasingly in medical practice they will need to be used judiciously, and usually under the direction of a health professional familiar with their purpose and use.

REFERENCES

1. Murtagh, J. (1984) An aid to patient education. *Australian Family Physician*, *13*, 463-4
2. Carson, N.E. and Baker, B. (1987) A desk top system. *Australian Family Physician*, *16*, 48-9
3. Leach, M.L. and Carson, N.E. (1985) Computerised drug information system for general practice. *Australian Family Physician*, *14*, 202-3
4. Shepherd Foundation. Health Risk Appraisal Program, 161 Fitzroy St, St Kilda 3182, Australia
5. Commonwealth Scientific and Industrial Research Organisation (CSIRO). Division of Human Nutrition, Kintore Avenue, Adelaide 5000, Australia
6. Baghurst, K.I. and Record, S.J. (1984) A computerized dietary analysis system for use with diet diaries or food frequency questionnaires. *Community Health Studies*, *8*, 11-18
7. Cohen, M. Sweetening diabetes education – computer-assisted instruction. (Submitted for publication)
8. Cohen, M. Diabetes Key Facts. Lions International Diabetes Institute, PO Box 185, South Caulfield 3162, Australia
9. Microcraft. Author, PO Box 63, Canterbury 3126, Australia

16

Information Technology and Public Health Education

Alan Maryon-Davis

FOR PEOPLE

Health education is a growth industry. Ten years ago it meant little more than sex lessons in school or posters on the waiting-room wall. Today almost every newspaper or magazine has a regular health feature; health items are a frequent ingredient of peak-time television; health education is woven into the typical school curriculum; and advice on smoking, alcohol intake, diet or exercise is increasingly earning a place as an important part of anticipatory care in general practice.

In schools teachers have for some years been able to use well-designed and field-tested teaching packs for education about smoking, diet, drugs or sexual responsibility. In adult educational settings such as the workplace there are 'off-the-peg' classes and courses for employees in, for instance, stress-management, sensible drinking or exercising. Health education materials have been specifically designed for use in the general practice setting, such as booklets to back up advice in the consultation, videos for patient groups, screening protocols for high-risk case-finding, and most importantly, training programmes for primary care professionals. And for the mass media there are briefing packs for journalists and producers, lists of expert contacts, and a high degree of collaboration between health educators and media professionals in the planning of programmes and articles. Health education is by definition all about providing information and developing skills to use that information effectively to promote health.

And yet, surprisingly for an industry based on information, health education has been slow to harness the enormous potential of new information technology. In its many and various settings it has been reluctant to explore alternatives to such traditional media as direct face-to-face teaching, either individually or in groups; the printed word in the form of leaflets, booklets and posters; audio-visual resources such as slides, films, audiotapes and videotapes; and the traditional mass media of newspapers, magazines, radio and television. It is only very recently that computer-based information technology (IT) has started to play a significant part in public health education. But after a somewhat tentative beginning there are now some exciting prospects in the pipeline.

In Britain there have been two main applications of IT as a direct medium for health education, and each has been developed steadily, albeit slowly, over the past decade — they are videotex and computer-assisted learning (CAL).

Videotex

Videotex is the generic name for computer-generated text on television. First developed in the UK in the late 1970s, it comprises the following elements:

1. a central computer to store information, linked to . . .
2. a multiplicity of viewing screens, either TV or micro VDUs, displaying . . .
3. standard format, 40 column × 26 line, seven-colour, pages that are . . .
4. easily updated and user-friendly.

The three types of videotex currently in use are teletext, viewdata and cabletext. They differ in the way the information is distributed to the receiving terminals.[1]

Teletext

Teletext is the most widely known type of videotex system. Distribution of the information is via a broadcast television signal — BBC (Ceefax), ITV (Oracle) and Channel 4 (4-Tel) — producing pages of text and graphics on TV sets in the home. Teletext-receiving sets are specially adapted to decode the signal. The pages are broadcast in a rotating sequence, one after the other in numerical order. Viewers are initially presented with an index page from which they

213

can select the number of the page they want using a remote control selector. This page is then 'captured' and displayed on the screen.

Teletext has been mainly used for providing information on such popular themes as the weather, travel news, recipes, gardening hints and share prices. But it has also conveyed information supplied by the Health Education Council on topics such as giving up smoking, healthy eating, infant immunisation and sensible drinking. Recently teletext has been used to disseminate software ('download' programs) to individual microcomputers in homes and schools. This application has great potential for health education (see below).

Viewdata

Viewdata is computer-generated text sent to TV screens via the telephone line, using a special adapter called a 'modem' and an inputting keypad. British Telecom's viewdata service has the tradename Prestel, and its great advantage over teletext is that it is interactive; the user can communicate with the central computer so that information is two-way. Successive pages are accessed by selecting from a series of 'menus' which guide the user through the data base algorithm. Information on Prestel is currently provided by about 200 different organisations. In effect Prestel works more like a bookstall than a publisher. It creates the vehicle for the information providers, but is not responsible for the accuracy of the data it carries.

Prestel has been used extensively for health education. The Health Education Council was one of the earliest information providers, with pages on healthy eating, exercise, immunisation, sensible drinking and advice on how to give up smoking. A list of HEC free publications was provided with instructions on how to obtain them. Other organisations, such as the Consumers' Association and the DHSS, have also provided health information.

There are two particular features of Prestel which extend its use in health education. Firstly, because it can be programmed to demand a password, it can be used for 'closed user groups', i.e. private networks. For example, the HEC set up a closed user group for health education units throughout the country, which has been used to provide information on forthcoming publications, conferences and campaigns, and facilitate ordering of bulk supplies of leaflets and posters.

Secondly, the user's terminal can be linked with other data bases via the central computer. In other words, Prestel can be used as a 'gateway' to a whole range of specialist sources of information, with which the user can interact. This is the basis of such computerised services as travel booking, home-banking, tele-shopping and accessing 'libraries' of software to download off-the-peg programs.

Since 1985 Prestel has been running a service aimed specifically at schools — Prestel Education. The service acts primarily as a resource for teachers in schools and higher education, not only as a direct source of information but also by distributing down-the-line software for computer-assisted learning.[2] The HEC has provided Prestel Education with information on smoking, nutrition, exercise, substance abuse, sex education and many other health education topics.

Cabletext

This is a combination of broadcast and down-the-line videotex. A number of parts of the country have been 'wired' for cable TV, and several services are being run currently on an experimental basis. The choice of channels for such services has been greatly increased with the advent of satellite TV, beamed to a central dish and distributed via cable to homes, offices and schools. Cabletext magazines, such as British Telecom's Skytext, are being developed for broadcast on satellite services. On a smaller scale, networked microcomputers or word processors, for example in the same office building, can be provided with a private viewdata service, generated entirely within the organisation and tailored to its particular information needs. Such networks have been shown to be an effective means of health education in the USA.[3]

So what opportunities does videotex offer health education for the future? The advent of satellite and cable TV will mean many more TV channels at relatively low cost, each capable of carrying videotex. Cable in particular, using optical fibres to relay the signal with the twin advantages of massive carrying capacity and freedom from interference, will be able to offer a much greater choice of videotex services to subscribers. Optical fibre will also revolutionise viewdata services, such as Prestel. The capacity to carry much more information will mean a greater use of computer-generated graphics and animation blended in with the text. We can expect to see a much greater range of videotex specifically for health education; some designed for schools, some aimed directly at the general public and some providing a resource for the many professionals involved in health education.

Computer-assisted learning

Perhaps the most notable development in teaching over the past decade has been the use of microcomputers as an aid to instruction. This computer-assisted learning (CAL) was given a major boost in the early 1980s by the government-sponsored Microelectronics Education Programme for schools, coupled with the advent of inexpensive hardware such as the Acorn/BBC micro, purpose-built for use in schools. The result has been a proliferation of well-tested CAL software, including health education programs.

The essence of CAL is that it is interactive, asking the learner a series of questions and responding appropriately to the answers given; thus leading the learner through an algorithm, or decision tree, of factual information or skills training.

However, there is much more to it than that. Most programs involve a blend of text and graphics, and much use is made of games and simulations. For children the best CAL software is usually fun, not to say addictive. There are programs on human biology, nutrition, smoking education, road safety, home safety and many others, some of which rival the video arcades for holding children's attention. CAL is a joy for the shy child who is held back in class either by fear of looking foolish or difficulty relating to the teacher. The programs are always gently encouraging and unflappable, and the pupil gets instant feedback and can work at his/her own pace. The main disadvantages are that teaching is based largely on the written word, and that some pupils may experience 'technophobia'; difficulty coping with the computer's commands.[4] Both may be helped by the advent of user-friendly speech recognition and voice production software; so that pupils can actually talk to the computer without having to rely on keyboard and screen.

Far fewer CAL programs are available for adults, largely because relatively few adults have access to a microcomputer. Those programs that do exist are used mainly for specific training purposes, e.g. fitness training, first-aid techniques, information for diabetics, etc. But as more people become micro users, more programs are being developed, many of them making use of some form of self-assessment as an indirect means of health education.

Self-assessment software

Providing information is only part of the business of health education — a much greater challenge is to get people to act on it. Motivation is the name of the game, and one of the best ways of achieving this is to 'personalise' the information, making it especially relevant to the persons concerned so that they feel to some extent that they 'own' the information and are therefore more inclined to act on it.

This is the principle behind the computer-based health self-assessment programs. The users are questioned about various aspects of their health or lifestyle and the computer builds up a profile which can be used as a benchmark to monitor changes. These changes might be in knowledge or attitudes about certain health concerns, health-linked behaviour such as smoking or exercise habits, or physical characteristics such as bodyweight or fitness parameters. Perhaps the most widely used type of self-assessment software comprises the many multiphasic health-risk appraisal programs particularly popular in the USA.

Health-risk appraisal (HRA) is simple enough in principle. An individual's health-related lifestyle is compared with norms derived from epidemiological and other data in order to assess his/her relative risk of developing or dying of such disorders as heart disease or cancer. An attempt is made to quantify such excess risk, either in terms of life expectancy or likelihood of disease, and to relate this where possible to specific behaviours, e.g. smoking, lack of exercise, unhealthy diet. Based on this assessment, a prescription for behaviour change is given, together with personal targets to be achieved within stated time limits.

Despite deficiencies in the various methods used to calculate risk, HRA programs have been found to be an effective means of conveying information about health-risk-related behaviour and to provide a useful stimulus to take action.[5] Self-assessment programs focusing on particular aspects of health, such as eating, drinking or exercise habits, have similarly proved successful, the two most popular types being those that deal with slimming and fitness.

Computer-generated graphics

Traditional health education techniques such as the use of leaflets and illustrated talks have been given a boost by new technology, particularly by new graphics software. High-quality visual teaching materials such as slides and overhead projector gels can now be produced from computer-generated graphics. Graphs, bar charts and pie charts can be instantly plotted from raw data, and other software can 'paint' diagrams and pictures; again useful for visual presentations. Such graphics can now be integrated with word-processed text, and whole pages can be designed in a variety of formats. The technique, dubbed 'desk-top publishing', is menu-driven and user-friendly, making the production of hand-outs, fact-sheets and leaflets both simple and cheap.[6]

Interactive video

One of the most exciting developments in information technology is the use of videodisc as an interactive educational tool. Known as 'interactive video' or IV, it combines the processing power of the microcomputer with the immense data storage capacity of the laser videodisc, resulting in a highly flexible and responsive teaching resource. Laser discs, normally used to reproduce television pictures, can store still pictures and other graphics as well as text. Their capacity is enormous; the entire contents of the *Encyclopaedia Britannica* will fit easily onto a single 12-inch disc.

The full teaching potential of IV has yet to be realised, but a fascinating glimpse was seen recently with the BBC's Domesday Project, in which a vast number of maps, photographs, tables, charts and sections of text, describing virtually every geographical location in the country, has been put onto a single laser disc, and digitally coded so that each item can be accessed almost immediately by an attached microcomputer using the Domesday software. The result is a mammoth compendium of data about Britain today, with which the user can call up a town or village, display a map of it, show pictures of the high street, church or pub, and show tables of population, local industries, etc. This sort of approach would lend itself very well to learning about the basic anatomy and physiology of the human body.

Hardware for reproducing 12-inch laser discs is expensive, as indeed are the discs themselves, but the recent popularity of compact discs (CDs) for audio reproduction has turned attention to the potential of CDs for IV use. Although current technology only allows CD discs to reproduce faithfully about 10 minutes of moving video (not enough to be a commercially viable proposition at present) they can still hold a massive amount of data as a read-only memory (ROM), enough for thousands of pages of text and hundreds of graphics. A CD player can be easily adapted to read text and graphics, and be linked to a microcomputer which, with appropriate software, provides the ultimate learning machine.

In early 1986 the Department of Trade and Industry set up the National Interactive Video Centre in London, a £1m three-year project to trial and evaluate the use of interactive video in schools. The Centre has produced a number of programs on a variety of subjects including biology, and results have so far been most encouraging. To date only one health education program has been trialled in this country, a program on alcohol education produced by the Health Education Council, but it is early days yet and more programs are in the pipeline. Certainly evidence from the USA suggests that CD-ROM is going to be the next great leap forward in educational technology and, combining as it does the properties of videotex, computer graphics, CAL and video, the potential for its use in health education is enormous.[7]

This potential would be enhanced still further if the CD disc could be written on as well as read from: being currently a type of read-only memory (ROM). Technology is halfway to this goal with the use of a small high-powered laser to burn microscopic pits on a reflective surface. These pits cannot be erased, but the capacity of the disc is so huge that new data can be added continuously and redundant data can simply be ignored. Some sort of truly erasable optical system (read and write) remains just over the horizon, but when it arrives it will revolutionise educational technology.

Imagine being able to switch on your cable TV, select one of 50 channels being broadcast via satellite to your central neighbourhood dish, and download a whole CD full of software using your read'n'write CD drive. Then off you go for a picnic in the country, taking with you your lap-top flat-screen micro with speech capability, integrated CD drive and your newly written CD disc. And there in the corner of a cornfield, you utter a few commands and open up a whole world or words and pictures about how to avoid stress. Now that's the future of health education for you!

REFERENCES

1. Council for Educational Technology (1985) *Videotex*. CET Information Sheet No. 10. CET, London
2. Council for Educational Technology (1985) *Prestel Education Service and The Times Network for Schools: a comparative guide*, CET, London

3. Grunder, T.M. and Garrett, R.E. (1986) Interactive medical telecomputing: an alternative approach to community health education. *New England Journal of Medicine*, *1*, 982–5

4. Feldman, R.H.L., Hollander, R.B. and Rezmovic, V. (1986) Overcoming technophobia: the joys and anguish of computers in health education. *Health education*, *1*, 45–6

5. Victor, C.R. (1986) *Computerised health risk appraisal: a critical review*. Working Paper No. 1. Nottingham University Department of Community Medicine and Epidemiology

6. Rogers, G.W. (1985) Computer graphics: the state of the art. *Journal of Audiovisual Media in Medicine*, *8*, 14–18

7. Wertz, R.K. (1986) CD-ROM: a new advance in medical information retrieval. *Journal of the American Medical Association*, *256*, 3376–8

Part 5

Challenges for the Future

17

Computers in General Practice — the Future

David Metcalfe

From being a far-fetched idea in the early 1970s, computers as a real tool in ordinary practice are now generally accepted. At first the question was 'What could it possibly do?'; then it was 'But how could we afford it?'; later it was 'What sort?' and then 'When should we move?'. Any practice which has not installed a computer, or is not actively considering getting one, is slipping behind. GPs are either on top of their practices or underneath them, and apart from personal commitment, information control is the most important tool for being, and staying, on top.

A typical practice has three principals and 6300 patients, does 22,050 consultations, makes 1323 referrals, of which 400 result in admissions, prescribes 37,800 items, and orders 992 laboratory tests: *and is unlikely to be able to produce any of that data as a basis for planning, audit, or teaching*! Any small business with that sort of turnover which did not know more about its customers and its transactions would soon fail, if it did not fall foul of company law first. The GP who is on top of his or her practice maximises practice income, minimises administrative chores (so that practice administrative staff get greater job satisfaction), provides proper preventive coverage for the practice population, proper surveillance of patients with chronic disease, and therefore generates his or her own job satisfaction. A computer can help in each of those areas.

COMPUTER DEVELOPMENT

But the computers already installed are not even the Model T Fords of computing: they are the turn of the century Daimler Benz, the cars preceded by the man with the red flag!

Proportionally, the advances in computing in the past 10 years are analogous to the advances in motoring in 90! Similarly they have advanced from being the toys of the very rich to a taken-for-granted appendage to most households (whereas thankfully the driving age has remained at 17, pre-school children have shown themselves adept at computing, and many a struggling father has been pushed away from the keyboard by a child who says 'let me do it Dad . . .'!). As well as the cataclysmic fall in prices (due to market expansion more than competition), there have been two major trends: from concentration of power in large mainframes to dissemination to networked micros; and from custom-written software to off-the-shelf software that can run on a variety of machines. The important thing to realise is that these trends will not come to a halt, but will continue for the foreseeable future at much the same pace. It is, however, important to recognise that this does not justify a retreat to what was the justifiable question of the early 1980s: 'Wouldn't it be better to wait a bit?'. This is because configurations already on the market have far more spare capacity (both in computing power and volume of memory) than earlier systems, as well as being able to accept 'add-ons', and because they will accept a wider assortment of software. To buy is no longer to cross the Rubicon.

CONSEQUENCES

What has in fact happened is that the systems now available, let alone those in the pipeline, have overtaken our thinking about how to deploy and employ them. It is as if we bought aeroplanes but only saw them as useful for taxiing around the airfield. Mostly, so far, we have only used them to do the jobs previously done manually in the practices of those eccentrics who pioneered age–sex indices, 'E' Books, and a plethora of logs, notebooks and card indexes in an effort to be on top of their practices. What else could we get out of them?

Computer systems are *meta-technology*. Perhaps the only two previous examples of comparable significance were the wheel, some time in pre-history, and the steam engine in the eighteenth century. Both were new technology which made possible tremendous advances in other technology and in social organisation. A hierarchy of major innovation can be traced from settled agriculture, which freed man from the uncertainty of hunter-gathering; the steam engine which vastly increased his muscle power; telephony, radio and television which extended his special senses; and now computers which enormously enhance that part of his thinking ability which depends on the recall and array of information, trend analysis and projection. Commerce and industry have been quick to grasp some of the potential of this meta-technology but medicine, as usual reluctant to learn from outsiders, is being left behind. We seem to be thinking of these fundamentally powerful tools as gadgets for improving the *status quo* (not that the status quo, as represented by some practices we could do without, couldn't do with a lot of improvement!). Why aren't we thinking of how to reorganise the practice round the computer, instead of how to get a computer to reproduce the jobs that can be done manually so that everything can go on as it was before?

CLINICAL MEDICINE AS INFORMATIONAL TRANSACTION

Clinical medicine is essentially an informational transaction: information is provided by the patient, processed by the doctor in terms of diagnosis and management plan, returned to the patient in its new configuration as a basis for negotiation and is recorded for a variety of purposes from trend analysis (management of chronics) through baseline data to quality control (audit) and legal safeguards. It is, however, seldom seen in these terms, but as a series of separate clinical tasks each with its own objective within the overall, but seldom explicit, goal of patient care: history and examination to establish the diagnosis; review of management options for efficacy, safety and acceptability; explanation and instruction in order to procure compliance; and a *post-hoc* diarisation of the event to provide an *aide-memoire* at the start of the next encounter. Described in this way the tasks can be seen to 'cone down', to reduce the information in use at each stage so as to simplify the task. For example, all the data from the history and examination can be jettisoned once they are subsumed by the diagnosis. This happens not only in the record (where the only entry might be 'osteoarthritis' whatever the site, duration, periodicity and physical signs), but to a considerable extent in the doctor's head (where once a 'diagnosis' has been achieved the evidence quickly fades: the patient is thought of henceforth, uncritically, as being osteoarthritic). There are, however, costs for this process: firstly that if the diagnosis is insecure the chance of review is lost (suppose it was really gout: was the joint hot?); and secondly the need to explain the diagnosis and plan to the patient in terms of his or her perceptions is frustrated.

COMPUTERS AND CONSULTATIONS

'Coning down' is in fact the only practicable way of doing the job 'in head', because we can only process a limited amount of information at any one time. A computer, on the other hand, doesn't need to cone down; it can keep a wide range of facts under review all the time, examine their interrelationships, and warn if any of these conform to critical criteria which it has been programmed to recognise. The doctor then doesn't need frantically to change focus between previous illnesses, occupational hazards, other medication, allergies and family history, not all of which will have been discussed at this consultation, but any of which may have a bearing on the nature of the problem and its management. He or she can respond to the patients' perceptions, interpretations and expectations, secure in the knowledge that 'background' linkages will be brought to his or her attention. Both doctor and patient have more 'space'.

'Space' is important. Being well means having plenty of personal space: having a wide range of choice, freedom to decide how to live your life. Space is diminished by illness, disability, pain, and by the psychosocial impact of poverty, rotten housing, unemployment and fear. It can also be diminished by insensitive health professionals, who may for the best of reasons try to control various aspects of their patients' lives. It is important to conduct the consultation in a way that protects or enhances the patients' space, so that they can work through their agenda, and feel comfortable about bringing very private, or very frightening, things out into the open. But the doctor needs space too: freedom from hassle, freedom from anxiety ('what might I be missing?), and from insecurity ('do I know enough about this condition to cope?'). The computer must subserve the consultation, not dominate it. It must be on call, not in charge. It must not get between the doctor and the patient, either physically or metaphorically, by intruding to demand attention. Is it possible to envisage a system that can transform the transaction from a sequence of operations each of which dumps the information essential to the previous one, however valuable, to one in which information is automatically rearrayed into the most productive formulation for the purpose in hand, and made available in manageable quanta logically presented? After all, most consultations are simple and straightforward, concerning minor illness, or well-understood chronic conditions in people well known to the doctor: you can get through most surgeries 'flying on automatic pilot', and without being seriously intellectually challenged. 'Who needs a computer to get in on the act? It will only slow me down.'

But how well do we do? What is the error rate? How can there be such wide variations in the pattern of care: we can't all be right? Is our prescribing safe (10 per cent of all hospital admissions are complicated by iatrogenic factors, as are 15 per cent of all inpatient stays) and economical? Why are 70 per cent of patients referred and found to have colorectal cancer at stage C, which has half the five-year survival of those picked up at stage A? Why do people with chronic diseases like diabetes have to traipse up to outpatients, to be seen by ever-different juniors, when we have both the clinical and personal knowledge to offer them proper surveillance. Ah, but do we have the clinical knowledge, or has it got a bit dusty? Keeping up to date is difficult: reading it up seems disconnected from the real world; what you learn at postgraduate sessions is better, but it is often a long time before you see a case of that, and by that time you've forgotten what it was the lecturer said . . . . Every time one does an audit, the gap is not between one's own criteria and those offered by the pundits, but between what one thinks one is doing and what one actually does. One has the best of intentions, but at the time it was more important to respond to the patient's distress, or the laboratory was closed, or there was no homatropine, etc. The responsibility of the computer is to close that gap, to issue reminders, to warn, or to provide useful technical data appropriate to that particular patient at that time.

As soon as we remodel the consultation round the meta-technology of the computer, paradoxically we have more freedom to respond personally, sensitively, and empathically to the patient as a person, because it will significantly reduce the uncertainty field in any transaction.

So what will such systems look like?

THE CHANGING CONSULTATION

The traditional consultation has always been a 'diadic' interaction between patient and doctor (Figure 17.1) characterised by a gross imbalance of power. (The doctor being of high social status, expert, healthy, on his own territory, and male: all characteristics of power.

COMPUTERS IN GENERAL PRACTICE — THE FUTURE

Figure 17.1: A diadic, traditional consultation

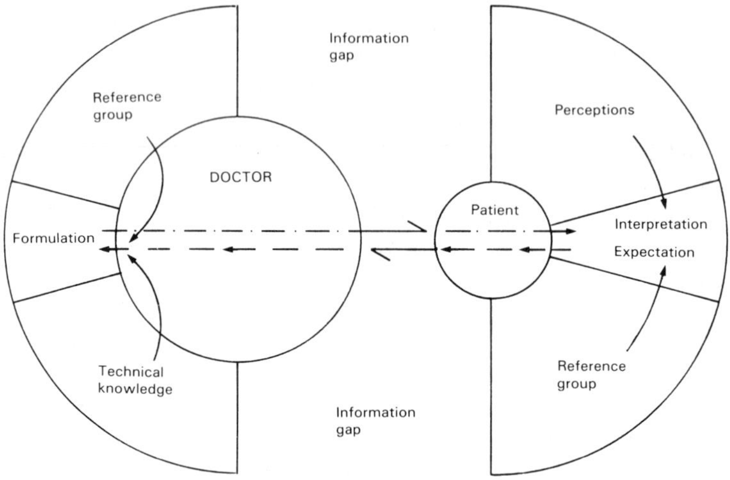

Reference group: the idea of how similar people to yourself would behave in similar situations

The patient is almost certain to be of lower status, inexpert by definition, poorly, off her own territory, and, because of higher consulting rates, female: circumstances pertaining to weakness.) Although we pay lip service to 'patient-centred medicine' this is difficult in a diadic interaction: the doctor cannot wrap himself round the patient. When, however, you add a computer to the transaction (Figure 17.2) the balance can change, provided that the patient has at least some access to the terminal, because by being able to do that she gains access to information, the stuff of power. She could see what is on her summary, or better still her Problem List (Lawrence Weed advocated patients agreeing to, and signing, their Problem Lists as the basis for a contract of care!), and correct it, or query it where necessary. She could ask for, and read for herself, data about the drug the doctor wants to prescribe. She could observe, and feel comforted by, the care with which her doctor used decision aids. Indeed there are already well-authenticated systems whereby patients use computer terminals to input their own health data

Figure 17.2: How addition of a computer changes the result

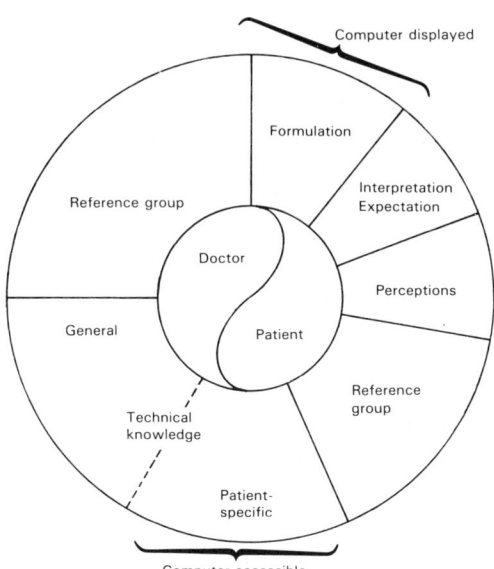

(whether previous illnesses, family history, occupational and housing data, etc; or 'sensitive' material such as information about psychosexual problems, where a terminal can be less embarrassing to talk to than some doctors). These data would be put in elsewhere and at other times, but could be accessed and reviewed in the consultation. At each phase of the consultation the doctor could 'cone down' as usual, confident that the screen would gently remind him, and the watching patient, about 'unfinished business' or intervening variables that should be kept in play. Far from exposing the doctor's frailties to the patient, this could be arranged in such a way as to enhance her trust in his thoroughness and care.

Of course both hardware and software would have to be designed to facilitate this sort of consultation. Screens must be easily readable, and data entry made as easy as possible, whether by two-letter codes, icons and the mouse, touch sensitive screens, or voice entry. GP input would have to be minimal: a brief entry to record presenting symptoms and critical signs, provisional diagnosis and management plan, to give the program enough to work on to apply its supporting review, with other services on call.

At the end of each episode the computer would automatically preen the record and dump any information which can, with that much hindsight, be seen to be subsumed in the statements such as the diagnosis, which of course would remain in the record. In this way volume of storage and search times could be controlled.

The narrative and summary record would, of course, not only serve the care of the individual patient, but would generate practice management tools such as the diagnostic index, therapeutic analysis and automated audits. It would be easy to indicate, either by the formulation of general rules, or case by case, what part of the record should automatically be inserted into referral letters.

Of course the office end, like the consulting room end, provides access to a variety of services already commonplace in commerce and industry, such as electronic mail and bulletin board services, access to data bases, etc. One wonders how long health authorities will be constrained to rely on typewritten letters sent to GPs through the post! Record entries, operation notes and laboratory results could be instantaneously transmitted to the patients' doctors as they become available, without a separate letter-writing process being added, with the concomitant delay.

This outline of a patient-centred, computer-serviced consultation draws attention to the central tenet of GP computers as meta-technology: that is that the system starts in the consulting room and spreads out to the office, rather than the consulting room terminals being outstations on tentacles from the office! A reversal of the present position.

18

The Health Care Paradox — Implications for Computing in Primary Health Care

Nigel Stott

The therapeutic paradox
Whereas the potential of medical knowledge for preserving and restoring health has never been greater and is still increasing, the systems for applying it have never been so sharply criticised.
Douglas Black, 1979

The preventive paradox
A measure which brings large benefits to the community offers little to the participating individual.
Geoffrey Rose, 1981

Fascination with paradoxes is not new. The 3000-year-old Chinese Yin and Yang represent a balance of opposites to produce health; the Bible is full of parables and paradoxes which help to reveal the true nature of man; Hegelian philosophy (1770–1831) deals with metaphysical contradictions and solutions from which Marx and Engels propagated the theory of dialectical materialism to explain political events by conflict between opposing social forces. Even modern physics has found itself immersed in paradoxes such as wave/particle theory. It can now be said that subatomic particles are both destructible and indestructible at the same time: because when two particles collide with high energies they can break into pieces which are not smaller than the original particles.

Paradox and truth seem to be as closely intertwined as the strands of DNA in a cell nucleus, and whenever we see a paradox arising from sound data it is likely that we are experiencing a tantalizing glimpse of one side of a great truth, which with further research or insight is only paradoxical when viewed from a blinkered position.

What does the law of paradox have to do with the implications of computers in primary health care?

The thesis I wish to develop is that computers have arisen from reductionist thinking, and they are having a growing impact on primary health care for better *and* for worse. As we look towards the future we can either simplify the possible scenarios to create a dichotomy between competing trends, or use the much more attractive and ancient law of paradoxical truth which states that it is impossible to live in a creative relationship with the world until everything is apprehended in relation to its opposite. Tension between opposites causes damage if the poles are viewed as independent of one another (a competitive destructive situation). If each person or each issue is viewed as a mixture of opposites in varying degree, then and only then can tension become truly creative and original.

Computers in family practice and primary health care are presently fulfilling a number of functions:

(1) They provide a sophisticated filing system, often from data of doubtful value. The old manual systems usually contained similar data, but made the data so inaccessible that they could not be used to draw individual or cohort conclusions.(Filing)
(2) They provide the means for increasing the amount of data collected in a compact space. The physical size of manual systems inhibits major expansion of data collection.
 (Size of data base)
(3) They provide statistical analysis power, thus permitting numeric and graphic representation of data of uncertain value to people who may now understand its limitations.
 (Statistics and management)
(4) They provide the means for quick mailing to some/all of the patients on the register, thus changing the relationships between doctor and patient with consummate ease.(Outreach)

These four functions are paradoxical in so far as each can be viewed as good or bad depending on the vantage-point of the viewer. Is it good to have greater analytic power or dangerous to draw conclusions from data which were not collected for hypothesis testing? Is it fair to have more data before the actors have agreed to their appropriate use? Is it good to recall people who are well, or could this in itself make them less well? Is it acceptable or unacceptable to store more personal information if the person involved has not agreed? Is it good or harmful to create dependence on a computer system? Is it possible that computerised records will help clinicians control patients or empower and involve patients more?[1]

Ethical, moral and practical problems surround these issues, but an important question remains: 'Is technology driving or serving clinical practice?' General practice computing seems to be riddled with the schemes of single-minded men who have succeeded within their self-defined framework of reference yet failed to comprehend the hazards of their systems. The paradox is that achieving a desired end may not be successful.

BALANCED PARADOXICAL COMPUTING

The tensions created by awareness of paradoxes in computing issues will assist many changes in primary health care. As soon as *all* data are viewed as clean *and* dirty, rather than as clean *or* dirty, it becomes possible to pose sensible questions and get more sensible answers with appropriate scientific humility about the conclusions. For example, an analysis of all children aged 5–15 years with the symptom label of 'sore throat' may be clean in symptom terms yet useless in aetiological terms; a sore throat may be socially determined or physically determined or both or neither; it may be symbolic or concrete or both or neither; respiratory or oral or both or neither; severe or trivial or both or neither. Suddenly the traditional biomedical approach becomes a very narrow focus and the breadth of primary health care unfolds in all its exciting and colourful manifestations; not least of which is questioning about the meaning of existing data.

All nosological systems both clarify and confuse. The very process of classification means ignoring some components of the context or environment or creature. As artificial intelligence is researched, and as computer systems become more sophisticated, they will become more and more like our brains: able to accept and deny the same information, to learn by context as well as by content, to see the correctness in an algorithm as well as futility in its specific application. Questions like 'Have you achieved a 100 per cent measles immunisation rate?' will be scorned as a crass and unethical oversimplification. A better question would well be 'What is the incidence of measles in your area and how do you interpret the data?' In one area 98 per cent freedom from measles is a huge success; in another 68 per cent freedom from measles is an even greater success because figures have meaning in individual contexts, and only brutal innuendos in isolation.

Money is perhaps the most insidious force operating towards the creation of opposites. The computing industry has been quick to use (or abuse) that component of man which is full of greed and fear. The pecuniary instinct is almost worshipped in some circles, so the promoters of most current microcomputing systems pander to it:

'Smears mean money — computers help'
'Screening increases practice income'
'Employ a nurse — it's cost-effective — and she will need a data base'

Such headlines in most editions of the popular medical press encourage polarity towards a cash flow mentality in a profession which likes to believe that the public have confidence in its ethical standards and moral uprightness. The paradox is that the headlines are true . . . and false. Also that each of us is ethical and unethical, sometimes at different times and sometimes at the same time.

The systems of the future will have to grasp the dangers of polarised dichotomies. As computer 'intelligence' begins to be more like human intelligence the duality in our natures and motives will be matched or near-matched. Truth is revealed by ambiguity and paradox, and it laughs at the pompous nonsense of polarised oversimplicity. When men believed the world was flat they could have programmed a computer to believe the same. Now we believe that the earth is round, are we capable of programming a machine which will, without internal stress, believe that both are true . . . and that both are false? Truth often depends on the context of perceptions. This may anger some people but, paradoxically, it is usually true.

When we accept that paradoxes often help to clarify truth we will have taken another step forward in science, art, technology and religion. However, my vision for medical computing is that it will continue to force us away from truth until we have really grasped the law of paradox for ourselves, and also learned the relevance of expert computer systems which will relate content to context.[2]

THE HEALTH CARE PARADOX

The health care paradox (or balanced ambiguity) states that it is impossible for doctors/nurses to live in a creative relationship with the public they serve until every discovery/observation has an understandable relationship to its opposite. Indeed, as I have said elsewhere,[3] 'Ambiguity is closely allied to balance because opposing forces can be in balance yet utterly ambiguous when considered from different viewpoints . . . the excitement, challenges and satisfactions in primary health care appear when an understanding of the biomedical meets the other half.'

Paradoxes lie at the heart of most creative thought, but they stop being stimulating when they have popular acceptance. One paradox which has not yet met with popular acceptance is the fact that few clinical problems have an unambiguous pathological basis. Biomedical assessments are therefore incomplete, yet the majority of data currently stored on health service records and computers is biomedical or administrative; like the least creative of human minds the computer will store these half-data and reproduce them.

Medical computing, which is constrained by reductionist and linear thinking, reveals only part of its potential. Real progress should emerge during the next decade as the importance of paradox becomes assimilated into current practice and planning. The transition for black-and-white thinkers is likely to be painful, but change is on its way and old-style algorithms will become as old-fashioned as the waterwheel. Biomedical purity will be more widely recognised as the part-truth it is now known to be by those who are able to grasp the law of paradox and to apply it with wholesomeness.

THE IMPLICATIONS FOR PATIENTS

The great advantage of having minimal recorded clinical data in old-style general practice is that the doctor conducts each interview within the framework of the presenting problem(s) and in the context of a variable, often impressionistic, recall of what has happened on previous contacts with the family. There is room for prejudice but this is offset by the human tendency to forget that which is less pleasant. Modern primary health care demands more detailed and specific recall for continuing problems, screening tests, lifestyle, acute problems and sociodemographic background. This 'data base' is deemed necessary for the practice of integrated, continuing and comprehensive primary health care.

The potential misfortune for the modern patient is that the new 'data base' is often de-personalised by being printed rather than

Table 18.1: Sample front sheet

Date	Problems	Date	Risk factors/promotion
1969	Dysmenorrhoea		
1976	TOP		Family history: Asthma Hyperthyroidism
1977	Pelvic inflammatory disease	1960	Rubella immune
		1970	Ex-smoker
1980	Infertility	1980	BP 120/80
1986	Marital problems	1984	Cervical smear normal
		1984	BSE learned
		1985	Smokes 20/day Alcohol 10-15 units/week

written, and placed in a prominent place in the record so what was discreetly semi-legible becomes data for every locum, trainee or partner to utilize. The printed word also has an aura of authority and validity. Consider the front sheet for a woman of 38 years in 1986, shown in Table 18.1. What a neat summary. At a glance any person with background clinical knowledge could infer causal linkages between the events in the problem list which could be quite erroneous. Likewise the chronological risk factor/promotion listing is bald data which is underpinned by a host of unrecorded human fears, feelings, experiences and expectations. Is her lifestyle adaptive or maladaptive?

The clinical paradox is that the data reveal so much, and hide even more. How doctors/nurses use such data in the clinical setting must be a source of concern to us all, because simplistic judgements based on the 'hard' biomedical information by one who may not have a continuing relationship and understanding with the patient is either dangerous or insensitive.

Understanding these issues may help clinicians to be cautious about using incomplete data to make premature inferences or judgements, but is that enough protection for the patient? The data system which reveals so much also has a responsibility to help the clinician comprehend the context of the data so in the haste of clinical work he/she is helped to be sensitive to issues which may modify interpretation of the same data. The future for patient-centred computing must be the linking of content to context; this will mean that bald data are qualified by why (?), how (?) or when (?), and visual images will have to complement the written word to aid conceptual understanding and avoid surplus text.

The alternative approach is to ensure that patients either keep their own records or routinely censure/edit the content of their doctor's records. There is fascinating scope for experiments in this field during the next decade. My patient, on seeing her summary (Table 18.1), requested that the entire problem list be erased so she 'could forget the past and start a new life without having doctors/nurses knowing more about her than she wished to recall for herself'.

The health care paradox can be paraphrased to state that doctors can only live in a healthy and creative relationship with their patients when 'having sensitive data' has been understood in relation to 'not having the same data'.

REFERENCES

1. Fitter, M. (1986) Evaluation of computers in primary health care. In: Peterson, H.E. and Schneider, W. (eds), *Human–computer communications in health care*. Elsevier, North Holland, pp. 67–80
2. d'Agapeyeff, A. (1985) The communication of knowledge. In: Bryant, J. and Kostrewski, B. (eds), *Current perspectives in health computing*. Bristol Computer Society, pp. 1–13
3. Stott, N.C.H. (1983) *Primary health care: bridging the gap between theory and practice*. Springer Verlag, Berlin

FURTHER READING

Black, D. (1979) The paradox of medical care. *Journal of the Royal College of Physicians, London, 13*, 57–65
Happold, F.C. (1968) *The Journey inwards*. Darton Longman & Todd, London, p. 84
Ritchie, L.D. (1984) *Computers in primary care*. Heinemann, London
Rose, G.A. (1981) Strategy of prevention: lessons from cardiovascular disease. *British Medical Journal, 2*, 1847–51
Snow, C.P. (1964) *The two cultures and a second look*. Cambridge University Press, Cambridge

19

Why Computerised Clinical Records are Indispensable

Bob Johnson

In 1986 more than half the office desks in the United States sported a computer. By 1990 fewer than one in four will be without.[1] The comparable figure for British general practitioners is likely to be less than one in 100, and not yet set to rise dramatically.* This chapter examines why this should be so, and what potential benefits are being lost as a result. How long it will take for the latter to coax such a computer desert into bloom is not easy to judge, involving as it does such non-electronic tangles as human inertia and whim, not to mention politics. Such topics fall well beyond the scope of this abbreviated review of mechanising general practitioners' clinical records.

The chapter falls conveniently into five sections as follows:

(1) costs – money
(2) costs – time
(3) computers compel codes
(4) Martindale digitised
(5) real prescriber support

COSTS — MONEY

Cost undoubtedly puts general practitioners off computing more than anything else, though Amstrad and others are set to change this. When I started medical computing in 1967 the machines in use sold

---

* This figure may be estimated from the fact that only 500–1000 practices have computers, say between 5 and 10 per cent of all UK surgeries. Of these, remarkably few have them on the consulting room desk.

for around £1 million. I shall never forget the temple-like structure that housed the computing equipment at Keele University in 1970. The white-coated acolytes who 'serviced' the machine were to be approached with a deference and decorum deriving entirely from the enormous capital costs invested all around them.

By 1974 a barely adequate machine could be had for £20,000. Even so, this was beyond the research resources of a single-handed general practitioner, especially when no other funds were forthcoming. The launch of the IBM-AT, in 1984, saw the first machine with sufficient capacity to do the job, and priced at below £5,000. In September 1986, Amstrad launched a series of IBM-compatible computers selling in the range £400–1000, perfectly adequate for most general practice computing.

It is important to appreciate what the wider factors are that propel this dramatic change. Some years ago *The Economist* carried a headline to the effect that since electronic computer circuits had fallen in price by 50 per cent every year for the past 20 years, those who waited long enough would be handed hardware for free; comforting advice for an unconventional computist.

As recently as July 1986 the prime memory chip, the 256 Kbit RAM, had fallen in price to $2, having been $100 only six months earlier.[2] Indications are that it will fall further to $1 in due course. A hundred-fold decrease in the price of its main building block in a matter of months must have a remarkable impact on the costs of computing in general.

Nor is the end yet in sight. Just as the 256 Kbit chip is replacing the earlier 64K version, so the 1 megabit chip is already on its way, with its successors lining up behind it. In due course the 1 megabit chip will be displaced by those capable of holding four million binary digits each, and in short order by those holding 16 million.

Since eight binary digits are required to store one character or byte, a million characters, or one megabyte would require 32 chips of 256 Kbits each. Current cost (July 1986) for one million characters of store is therefore $64, set to fall to $32 when each of the constituent chips halves in price. As more bytes are packed onto the same quantity of silicon, each megabyte will cost first $8, $2, then 50 cents as the price of each piece of silicon, regardless of its contents, falls to its irreducible minimum of $1.[3]

It is worth dwelling on this point, for it is the one area in this complicated topic where matters are becoming simpler and cheaper. Elsewhere more human factors come into play, which, as Browning[1] emphasises, play a larger part in this Data Revolution than they did in its Industrial predecessor.

One million characters is difficult to visualise. Estimates vary as to how much paper it represents, though it is safe to assume it would cover 400–500 sheets of A4, a pile some 50–100mm (2–4 inches) high. The price of 50 cents for such a quantity may seem a bargain, but these almost fairy-tale prices conceal a trap and a snare, into which the more gullible tumble without a second thought. Just imagine a book or (heaven forbid) a patient's record landing with a thud on the consulting room desk, with anything approaching a megabyte of information. The size of a double-length novel, it might never have been cheaper — but how long would it take to read?

The problem of reading through text does not go away simply because it has been laboriously typed onto pieces of silicon or stored on slivers of magnetic tape. For this, mere humans require the assistance of the electronic machine, else the data will go unread by busy practitioners. In order to enlist the help of these overgrown digital calculators the text must first be digitised. Justifying this statement is the burden of this chapter.

Reasons why general practice computing has had such a chequered commercial history have been much argued; but interested readers are referred to the excellent and, in my view, entirely realistic review by Tanner,[3] which deserves a wider circulation. Only pressures of space prevent me including it here.

Before leaving the question of financial costs it should be noted that the market forces which drive the electronics industry have recently begun to show signs of slackening. Browning[1] points out that annual growth rates among commercial computers has eased from 15 per cent down to 10 per cent. He also notes that 'Although computer hardware is falling in price by about one third each year, the demand for innovative software already outstrips supply.' The mention of software takes us onto the most costly element of computers.

COSTS — TIME

The computer desert that afflicts British general practice conceals further costs, less obvious than mere finance. The administrative and management structure of the NHS is such that one of the key resources a general practitioner must conserve, and dispense with greatest care, is time.

All computers, for all the microsecond speed of their internal switches, swallow inordinate quantities of human time, with hardly a blink of their mechanical eye. This was especially so for the pioneers, who would type for long hours in front of unforgiving VDUs, or for the earliest, at the card punch machine, the least merciful of all mechanical contrivances.

The question arises in acute form when the new computer system comes to be installed. How much of the past clinical histories already laboriously gathered, either on Lloyd-George cardboards, or the more voluminous A4s, should be typed into the system; and then, by whom.

The unfriendly digital computer has yet another trick up its sleeve. Not only can it swallow time, as if it was of no moment, it can do the same with text. The time penalty with computerising text comes not only with the typing in, but also with the reading out.

It is easy enough to skim through a book, 'just to get the feel of it', or to see if a particular item catches the eye. It is rather a different matter with a computerised data base. Doubtless as flat-screen technology progresses the actual electronic 'page' will come increasingly to resemble the comfortable and familiar paper page which we know so well. But the sheer size of the data base militates against any one item being easily accessible: the more there is, the more difficult it is to get at. This is 'data pollution'. To extract one item all its neighbours must be scanned by human eye. The time consumed is limited only by the attention span of the human operator.

This time penalty is a feature of all large data bases from libraries to telephone directories, whether computerised or not. It is a feature of all large collections of data, from which no textual data bank can escape. The data already there impede the retrieval of the selected item. Reading all the screenfuls of information in Martindale, On-line, for example would take a year.[4] Surely there must be a solution to this problem. If there is none, then the more assiduous the clinician in recording medical data, the more effectively is he or she burying that which has already been collected. Such a crippling data overload warrants exploring even unconventional solutions.

COMPUTERS COMPEL CODES

The digital machine manipulates digits with unimaginable speed and precision. Only by exploiting this digital feature can the problem of data pollution, or textual excess, be resolved. The data require first to be digitised or coded, not a popular proposition to date. But only a digitised data base can hope to solve the problem.

That digital computers perform best when fed digits might seem reasonable enough, except to those who believe that these incredible machines have yet more extraordinary facilities hidden up their silicon sleeves. Many man-years have already been spent struggling to humanise free text systems. The digital machine owes its very utility exclusively to the fact that it moves digits, especially binary digits, at astronomical speeds. It processes decimal digits and alphabetic characters less well; and words, phrases, and paragraphs not only with mastodonic slowness, but with illusions of accuracy. It is as if the machine moves simple light items fast, and complex cumbersome structures with a deadly sloth.

There are further hidden pitfalls. Human meaning is a fascinating, fluid and endlessly varied topic. Since earliest times attempts have been made to systematise, even to enumerate, it. Indeed, careful philosophical analysis over 30 years has happily culminated in an evaluation of the role of meaning in human affairs, and the subtle yet profound links that this has with that other human mystery, emotion. To be frank, without this philosophical framework to underpin the approach to digital computers offered here, this chapter would have faltered, even perhaps have foundered altogether. Much as the prospect tempts one, a fuller discussion of this point would take us well beyond the remit of this chapter. Interested readers are referred to a full account.[5]

Even to the most superficial observer, human nature must appear fickle, variable and imprecise. It seems to get along very well like that: but it takes most unkindly to being defined or tied into a machine.

A linguistic illustration will show some of the more obvious ramifications of the problem. One of the few medical conditions where the diagnosis can be close to 100 per cent certain, and ambiguities are least in evidence, is pregnancy. As it happens this is also a highly emotive human subject, and as such attracts an unusually large number of synonyms, allonyms, acronyms, allusive euphemisms and other linguistic and literary devices which, while delighting its human verbalists, utterly confound even the most persistent programmer.

A patient may describe any of the following symptoms: 'My period's late', 'My nipples have changed, and I have morning sickness', 'I missed the pill last month and I'm worried'.

Any general practitioners hearing or seeing written one of these symptoms would need to presume pregnancy until discounted. The prospect of writing a program that would instruct the computer to recognise the full significance (or meaning) of any and all of these lines should daunt even the most foolhardy. Humans enjoy variety in their discourse. Computers do not. To inflict the features of the latter on the former is not only discourteous, but smacking as it does of the totalitarian state will, in the longer run and in democratic societies, fail.

Clinicians are expected to diagnose; but, being also human, they record their diagnoses with variety if not ingenuity. They may use any of the following phrases:

'pregnant', 'pregnancy', 'cyesis', 'grande multipara', 'gravida 1', 'slide agglutination positive', 'primigravida', 'l.m.p.: 7 weeks, e.d.d.: 33 weeks', 'multipara', 'primipara'.

As with the symptom list given above, any one of these entries could easily find itself standing alone in a hastily written general practice medical record. Despite the cryptic nature of some of them, each would need to be thoroughly checked and verified before the diagnosis of pregnancy could be dismissed. It may be noted that there is a wider choice of phrase in the diagnostic category than with the symptoms. The responsibility for this rests entirely with the human physician recording the history. Having closer access to that record, the recorder has greater scope to allow his or her literary facilities free expression.

Some restriction on the form and range of input is clearly obligatory, otherwise the computer would spend all its time unravelling the verbal tangles in which we humans delight. But halfway houses such as limited vocabularies and 'permitted' lexicons impose discomfiting restrictions without unleashing the full digital processing power of these speedy machines.

A brief digression into data base structures is warranted here. The standard model, evolved gradually over many years, is the hierarchical or pyramidal data base: access is always and only from the top. The 'tree' model of 'directories' in P-DOS follows this pattern. This type of data base has only one entry point. That is to say all queries to the system must start from a single point – the so-called root directory. Movement within the data base is either up and down, or, at one level only, from side to side. This is obviously a cumbersome and slow structure, which is nevertheless relatively simple to program, and is therefore quite widespread and reliable.

More recently relational data bases (for a recent description see Cornes[5]) have increased the flexibility of these rigidly determined machines, by allowing access from several points. But as before, the basic data are still stored as free text, and are therefore unavailable for mechanical analysis.

Though there are now several points from which analysis of the stored data can be approached, there is still the problem of the precision and accuracy of the indices which lead the user to it. Again, once the target data have been found, they must still be read through 'manually', since they are stored as free text. Here again, the more data stored, and therefore the more comprehensive the data base, the greater the impedance to the user, and the slower does his or her overall progress become.

The ultimate computer data base is one which increases the number of entry or access points to their logical limit, that is so that every data item stored is accessible for computer manipulation. This requires devising a new numerical language, such as Medol (one of the Lingol group of languages). This permits the development of the digitised data base. This digression is necessarily brief; more general descriptions appear elsewhere.[4,6] The concept of dynamising the data base may be a difficult one to grasp, but its implications are profound.

MARTINDALE DIGITISED

The problems of entering records directly in digits is not as forbidding as might at first appear. The advantages are also more immediate, as a look at Martindale On-line will show. Martindale is perhaps the most important computerised data base yet to emerge. Table 19.1 shows a sample screenful produced in response to a search on 'vodka'. This screenful was distributed at the Primary Health Care Specialist Group's Oxford Conference, 1985. I assume it was selected since it achieved only one 'hit'. More hits would have overloaded the communication channel being used at that time, namely a single sheet of A4 paper.

Note that in order to extract the useful clinical information it is necessary to read through each of the lines in turn. This may not be very surprising, it is what human beings have always had to do since Babylonian times, when pages took the form of clay tablets, or sheets of papyrus. But when there are 18 megabytes of data, as with Martindale, the reading time consumes 12 man-months. Few

Table 19.1: A sample screenful from Martindale On-line

Search on: VODKA
1 hit
2679/a1/17-c
Paracetamol. Adverse Effects. Abstract.
Effects on the liver. Hepatotoxicity occurred in two patients who took up to 5 or 6.5 g of paracetamol daily for several weeks and in one patient who took about 3 g of paracetamol and drank one pint of VODKA daily for several years.
Barker-J-D, et-al.
Ann intern Med., 1977, Vol. 87, P: 299.7
Keywords PARACETAMOL, AE, LIVER-DISORDERS, LIVER, AD, ORAL-ROUTE.
Jan. 1983   441 characters

general practitioners have this sort of time available. Theirs is the greatest need for the clinical data lodged within Martindale, theirs too is the most pressing need for mechanical help in scanning through this vast and often-times vital treasure trove.

The coding system advocated has already been presented elsewhere,[7,8] and space precludes greater detail here. Besides, being a practical procedure it is vastly more simple to demonstrate in practice than to describe in cold print. For those interested, a demonstration disc is available to run on IBM-compatible machines. Before those sceptical of this approach dismiss it out of hand, perhaps they should try out this disc and see for themselves: all that is required is access to an Amstrad or equivalent, and half-an-hour's 'hands-on' experience – it would settle no end of arguments. Meanwhile a brief review is in order.

Table 19.2 shows the main structure of the Medol system. Each item can be broken down to ten further subdivisions, and then to perhaps another 100 each. In this way up to 1 million separate symptom codes become available, each related back to the simplicity of the 16 general codes shown. No code need ever be memorised, since all are displayed on the screen as needed, and none is stored until the recorder is entirely happy with what appears, in English, alongside the digits entered.

The objective is to satisfy the demands of the digital computer, namely that clinical data be digitised, while at the same time making the unnatural process as congenial as possible. In use, common things occur commonly, and over 80 per cent of all symptoms require no more than a score of these two-digit codes. 'Cough' at 'S21', for example, occurs on average three times a working day,

Table 19.2: The 16 general symptom codes

'System' (physiological)		'Reaction'	'Area' (anatomy)
		R10 pains	A10 head
S20 respiratory	(26%)		A20 chest
S30 mental	(21%)		A30 arm
S40 alimentary	(18%)	R40 'better'	A40 trunk
S50 skins, trauma & locomotory	(18%)	R50 'no change'	A50 leg
S60 genito-urinary (of which S65 pregnancy)	(10%)	R60 'worse'	
S70 ear, nose, eyes & metabolic	(4%)		
S80 cardio-vascular, neurological & allergy	(3%)		

(% = frequency of occurrence in decade of general practice)

and 'pain' at 'R10' four times daily, so it does not take long before one can enter either almost 'blindfold'.

Writing in numbers is an uncomfortable human activity. It has not been easy to persuade colleagues of its utility. But since the exigences of the digital machine, in my view, demand it, it seems prudent to make the best of a bad job, and 'humanise' the numbers as much as possible. The parts of the body shown in Table 19.2 under 'Area' are virtually self-explanatory. Simply entering a '10' under 'Reaction' and a '20' under 'Area', records the presence of pain in the chest. Substituting any of the other 'Area' codes allows the location of the pain in any conceivable part of the body.

In practice, I suggest, the system is much easier to use than to describe. I recorded all symptoms, diagnoses and treatments from August 1970 to February 1981, when only lack of funding compelled me to desist. I recorded 200,000 symptoms, with 140,000 treatments from 70,000 consultations. A compacted version of this digitised decade will shortly be available on an IBM-compatible disk for those interested in pursuing a variety of analyses. Confidentiality will, of course, be maintained.

Once digitised the digital machine really comes into its own. An Esperanto version, for example, of the entire ten-year data base is already well in hand. Less precise languages may be added later. Even the most elementary programmer can see how simple it is to pull out all references to chest pains, merely by scanning for all A20s preceded by an R10, a pain frequently of vital significance.

WHY COMPUTERISED CLINICAL RECORDS ARE INDISPENSABLE

'21–10–20' conveys 'cough with pain in the chest'. Adding the duration column, as in '21–10–20–1W' allows the recording of length of time the symptom has persisted. Moving rather abruptly from these simple fundamentals, let us examine how Medol would cope with Martindale's clinical data.

The clinical data given in the Martindale screenful above amount to:

> Effects on the liver. Hepatotoxicity occurred in two patients who took up to 5 or 6.5 g of paracetamol daily for several weeks and in one patient who took about 3 g of paracetamol and drank one pint of VODKA daily for several years.'

As text, this requires much storage, is difficult to handle inside the machine, and must be visually scanned by each human user who hopes to benefit from it. Some indication of the difficulty the machine has in digesting text is given by the fact that the programming structure required to accommodate 18 megabytes of drug data rises to 250 megabytes, a ratio of scaffolding to valuables of almost 1 : 14. It's like building the Eiffel Tower with kitchen tiles.

Suppose for each of the clinically important items in this text the machine had only a number or series of digits. The situation is then transformed. Not only do they require a twentieth of the storage (say two megabytes instead of 18), but they can be scanned through for whatever item the clinician might currently want. The technique for scanning for chest pains has already been mentioned. The same principles apply to every other clinical item, as the illustrative 'digitisation' in Figure 19.1 shows. The Medol screen showed these data after entering the details given in the text about the first patient. Already more accuracy is required than is available from the text: a given dosage has had to be assumed to cover the range given. The age and sex were excluded from Martindale owing to pressures of space. Only two extra bytes would suffice to put them in the digitised record.

Figure 19.1

	PATIENT ONE
3 3712 500 1 4 6	TREATMENT paracetamol 500mgs 3 tablets four daily for six weeks
1 0 37 9 0	REACTION to drug connected with
1 9 52 43 0	connected with hepatotoxicity upper abdomen

247

Medol works by typing in numbers only from the numeric key pad, which are then instantly translated on the screen, for the recorder to verify, and edit as required. Only numbers are entered, since this is what the computer will store, but words appear associated therewith, so that the human element can ensure that what goes in is what was intended.

The Medol record consists solely of the column of digits appearing on the left-hand side in Figure 19.1. Each of these is entered by the coder; the text appears automatically and without further coding action.

The '3' on the first line of code is thus a 'Treatment' line, as indicated by that word appearing automatically to the right of the digits. The drug code happens to be '3712', being paracetamol, but any numerical coding system could be substituted here, providing it was easy to use, and unambiguous. The strength of the tablets is covered by the '500', to be taken at the rate of three tablets four times a day for six weeks, the numbers simply being transliterated as shown. This odd dosage has been chosen to ensure a daily dose of six grammes, as specified in the text, The superior accuracy of the digitised record has entailed some 'invention'.

The second line of digits starts with a '1' to indicate symptoms, the most frequent item in the Medol system. R37 represents drug reaction reported by patient. The '9' under 'Area' stands for A09 which is used to connect two lines of code together, thus linking the drug reaction with hepatotoxicity. The A43 in the third line normally stands for upper abdomen. When 'modified' by R51 it signifies 'liver', and by R52 'hepatotoxicity'.

Again the details of the coding process come readily to hand on the screen: no single code need be memorised, though common ones become second nature very quickly (see Figure 19.2). The element of repetition shows up well, indicating the consistency of the digitised output regardless of the variability of the vocabulary in which the clinical input is expressed. The second line of the third patient shows how clinical details can be squeezed into the rigid digital structure. '1–03–82–83–3–3' conveys in sequence, a symptom (1), a modifier (S03) meaning 'much', a further modifier (R82) 'alcohol' being the second subdivision of (A83) 'to socialise'.

Then follow 3 units of 'years' to give the line 'much drink socialise 3 years'. This is rather poor English for 'drinks a pint of vodka a day for 3 years', which in itself is a further diminution of 'drank 1 pint of VODKA daily for several years'. The English may not be pristine, but the clinical meaning is fairly obvious; at least it

Figure 19.2

```
                        PATIENT TWO
3 3712 500 1 5 5   TREATMENT paracetamol 500 mgs 2 tablets
                   four hourly for 5 weeks
1 0 37 9 0         REACTION to drug connected with
1 9 52 43 0        connected with hepatotoxicity upper abdomen
```

```
                        PATIENT THREE
3 3712 500 1 3 6   TREATMENT paracetamol 500 mgs 2 tablets
                   three daily for 3 years
1 3 82 83 3 3      much drink socialise 3 years
1 0 37 9 0         REACTION to drug connected with
1 9 52 43 0        connected with hepatotoxicity upper abdomen.
```

is unambiguous. This would seem to be a reasonable price to pay for the benefits of digitised data.

A more serious point is the veracity of the data. Here the utterly unfathomable skill of 'taking a clinical history' comes into play. Humans learn to perform this indefinable activity as if it were second nature. Clinicians learn to extract items of clinical value from the infinite range of verbiage available to the patients who seek their help. Computers will never do this, because their human programmers cannot assemble a sufficiently clear account of precisely what transpires in the infinitely mysterious phenomenon of two human beings relating together.

What the Medol system does is neatly by-pass a morass of flailing linguistic philosophies, and takes what the doctor says the patient said as being gospel. It leaves the clinical process intact in its fascinating mysteries, and merely replaces the doctor's pen with a numeric keyboard. Other advantages follow.

Clinical judgement is an obscure mental process. It will always remain so. But the problem of data pollution in clinical records and drug data base does have a solution.

REAL PRESCRIBER SUPPORT

In its present form Martindale On-line is inaccessible to the average general practitioner who, being the highest prescriber in the NHS, is most in need of it. It is inaccessible, and will remain inaccessible for two reasons, both of which have been mentioned. Firstly 250 megabytes of program are difficult to accommodate, and being a complicated man-made product the system is liable to faults, apart from being decidedly expensive to set up, maintain and operate. Secondly, in terms of time the human visual system is simply not designed to read megabytes of data delivered at speed, in textual form.

The proof of these statements awaits the practical implementation of a digitised drug data base with the comprehensive value of Martindale. Meanwhile, Medol indicates a method of proceeding. Once drug information has been digitised or Medolised, then access to the actual data becomes not only fast, but precise. The computer itself can be deployed to scan through several megabytes 'in real time', that is to say fast enough to influence practical situations, in this case the prescribing of a new drug, by a busy general practitioner.

Suppose from the above illustration that you were about to prescribe paracetamol for a patient with whose previous history you were unfamiliar. His or her entire clinical history, once Medolised, could be carried by the patient with ease within the 16 Kbytes of a credit card-sized 'smart card'. 16 Kbytes cover 400 average patient/years records. This would be fed into your desk-top computer, and every item in it compared with the up-to-date drug date file already resident.

The drug data file would already have been digitised as above. The entire digitised Martindale data base, for example, would occupy only one-twentieth the storage of the text version. The computer then faces the task first of screening two million integers for the occurrence of say '3 3712' representing 'paracetamol' and then of screening some 16,000 integers for '1 03 82 83' representing excess alcohol consumption, as described above. 'Hits' would be displayed on the screen when and only when needed.

In computing terms this problem is as straightforward as finding pains in the chest. Computers operate best with digits, and subtracting one from another to see if they are identical can be accomplished two or three million times a second. The latest IBM, the RT (priced at around £8000) for example, is rated at 25 MHz, which could accomplish the above with ease, readily screening through two megabytes of numerical data in one second.

The textual alternative, in computing terms, is prohibitively difficult. Imagine having to keep track of the vocabularies of multiple human compilers of the drug data base, the clinical history, to say nothing of the memories of the patient or clinician. The point is best made by a challenge issued in 1972: 'However, while a clinician may resist the idea of writing a '1' and a '4' in the appropriate places, instead of his more familiar 'A, B, D, O, M, I, N, A, L, space, P, A, I, N': it does not necessarily follow that he will continue to do so, in the face of superior medical data processing.[9]

Response to this challenge has been conspicuous by its inaudibility: yet computer technology has made it yet more pertinent than when first issued. The astronomic quantities of medical data that seem likely to arrive before the end of this century merely adds further, and I would have thought inexorable, weight.

A global total of one trillion (10^{12}) symptoms seems probable between now and AD 2000.[8] Without computer assistance this will remain merely a data mountain, and informed medical practice yet another victim of data pollution. Yet even this astonishing number of symptoms could be screened today, in the mind-numbing space of 17 minutes, using the Cray 2 supercomputer,[10] running at 1,000,000,000 instructions per second.

Only a digitised data base offers the slightest hope of dealing with an otherwise nightmarish quantity of medical data. Those who prefer to ignore it consign themselves and the patients whom they treat to an unnecessarily toxic medical ignorance. Medical ignorance may be acceptable to the former, though I believe less so to those whom treatment is intended to benefit. It is factors such as these which compel, ever more convincingly, the clinical indispensability of digitised records.

REFERENCES

1. Browning, J. (1986) 'Information technology', a survey, quoting Dataquest. *Economist*, 12 July, p. 5
2. Schofield, J. (1986) Microfile. *Guardian*, 17 July, p. 15
3. Tanner, S. (1986) Buyers guide. *Practice Computing*, June, 5, 4-5
4. Johnson, R.A. (1986) Quick cure for a data base dilemma. *Guardian*, 1 May, p. 13
5. Cornes, R. (1986) A beginners guide to normalising data. *Guardian*, 10 July, p. 16
6. Johnson, R.A. (1986) A better way to code? *Practice Computing*, June, 5, 17-19
7. Johnson, R.A. (1984) *EMOTION and the vital spark*. Published by Medol Systems, 171 Manchester Road, Mossley, Tameside, Greater Manchester OL5 9AB, (ISBN 0-9510207-0-6)
8. Johnson, R.A. (1986) Adverse reactions in ten years general practice, computer analysed. *Journal of the Royal Society of Medicine*, 79, 145-8

9. Johnson, R.A. (1972) Computer analysis of the complete medical record including symptoms and treatment. *Journal of the Royal College of General Practitioners*, 22, 655–60

10. Darling, D. (1986) Seymour Cray's Realcool supercomputer. *Guardian*, 10 July, p. 16

20

General Practice at the Crossroads

Mike Fitter and Bob Garber

INTRODUCTION

General practice appears to have arrived at a crossroads. In the past 40 years it has developed from the typical single-handed practice, often based in the doctor's own home, to the group practice, increasingly based in a health centre. General practice as a profession has taken its place as an equal partner alongside other medical specialties. The importance of *primary* health care as an appropriate and cost-effective means of maintaining and improving the health of the nation is also being increasingly stressed.

Yet today general practice is under review, and there is a lengthy agenda for discussion (as for example in the Government 'Green Paper', 1986, and the Social Services Committee's response, 1987). The issues at stake include recognised regional variations in health and of standards of care; lack of effective teamwork and co-ordination with related welfare services; a desire for more preventive health care, but the absence of a comprehensive strategy for achieving it; a recognition that prescribing costs account for the majority of expenditure in general practice, combined with a belief that savings could be made, but with no demonstrably effective methods for doing so; the absence of an agreed method of assessing performance in general practice; and increased concern that the service be accountable and responsive to the needs of patients.

Standing at the crossroads, these we believe are some of the concerns that will influence the direction that general practice takes over the next few years. In this chapter we will describe some of the lessons we have learned while studying a wide range of general practices over the past eight years. We will also try to outline some of the choices available to general practice, and to anticipate what some of the consequences may be, depending on choices made.

Our experience has been concentrated on the development and use of information systems in general practice. However, the development of information systems in general practice is inextricably linked to the development of general practice as an organisation. There is necessarily a symbiotic relationship between an organisation and its information and control systems. Before getting down to details we would like to make some observations.

Medicine is the archetypal profession, and has been identified as having the following characteristics:

1. a high degree of autonomy — for example the profession determines its own standards of education and training, and is relatively free from lay evaluation and control; and

2. a service orientation — a commitment to 'look after' the needs and interests of its client group.[1]

This high level of professional autonomy distinguishes doctors from most other occupational groups. As a consequence, doctors have had far more direct influence over the design and development of information technology than other groups, for example bank or office workers. Several GPs in particular have been 'pioneers' in the development of general practice computer systems. Being independent contractors they have had the motivation and the means (the freedom to choose how they develop their work, the ability to acquire new skills rapidly and the financial resources to support their ideas) to develop the technology 'their way'.

In comparison with independent and skilled workers in previous times, it may be worth noting that at the beginning of the Industrial Revolution craftsmen in the wool and cotton industries had a similar level of autonomy over the practice of their own trades, though over the past 200 years this has entirely disappeared as complex, but standardised, work processes and technologies have superseded traditional methods of production.

It is an interesting question, to an occupational psychologist as well as to the medical profession, whether similar changes will occur in the practice of medicine. Whilst doctors maintain control over the development of new technologies it seems unlikely they will 'rationalise' and 'deskill' their own work, but this may not always be the case. At the moment we perceive a strong belief that the design of any worthwhile GP computer system has required the close involvement of a medical practitioner. To date much of the development has resulted from the initiative of individual doctors developing systems for their own use, either on their own or in partnership with a software house. This has led to a plethora of GP computer systems, to some extent a sign of the 'not invented here' syndrome, but also a genuine reflection of the diverse priorities and organisational forms that currently exist in general practice.

Our interest in general practice from the perspective of occupational psychologists is with the *way* in which information systems are developed and used, and the *impact* that such developments have on the effectiveness of general practice and on the people involved.

Developments can be seen from the multiple perspectives of a range of 'stakeholders' — the groups that have an interest in the way that general practice changes. Clearly GPs themselves are a central group, and this chapter is addressed primarily to them. But other groups of stakeholders include other *service providers* (e.g. other members of the primary care team and employed staff), the *clients* (patients), the *service funders and administrators* (e.g. the DHSS and FPCs), and the *information technology promoters* (system developers and suppliers). The perspective and interests of each stakeholder group will be different, though probably overlapping.[2] One aim of research on the development of information systems in general practice is to *evaluate* the impact for each stakeholder group, and to *articulate* the likely consequences of further developments which are under active consideration. Before looking forward to the impact which computing may have on general practice in the coming years we will review some of the reported effects to date.

THE USE OF COMPUTERS IN GENERAL PRACTICE: WHAT HAVE WE LEARNED?

Today some 10 per cent of general practices in the UK have a microcomputer. Many of these have had their system for several years and acquired it through the Government-sponsored 'Micros for GPs' scheme. The Final Report on the scheme[3] concluded that progress in many of the 140 practices involved had been fairly slow over the first 12 months of computer use. Although the practices had learned from their own and others' experience how to introduce and use computers, and how to specify their computing needs more effectively, much was still to be done. The Report[3] also concluded that:

There is a growing awareness that as a rule the main benefits of computerization do not lie in the mimicry of manual procedures to carry out the routine tasks relating to individual patients — registration, repeat prescriptions, simple recall. Indeed it seems doubtful that the costs of computing can be justified on this account alone. Rather it is in the aggregation and analysis of information that the computer's analytic strengths seem to offer real advantages. However, an adequate assessment of the computer's value here requires a longer period than the 12 months use so far examined (p. 10).

Thus a further study was commissioned by the DHSS and reported in October 1986. This study followed up on 65 of the original practices some 30 months after they started using their computer, and also examined a further ten practices mainly from outside of the original scheme, but which had been identified as making particularly 'high use' of their computer.[4] The study examined how *extensively* and how *effectively* the computers were being used. It also looked at the views of the practice members (GPs and employed staff), and how they perceived the computer as affecting the practice and their work. In this latter area we are now studying the available data in more detail.

The computer in the office

The second study found that substantially more progress had been made than had been observed in the previous study, and most practices made extensive use of their computer for registration, repeat prescribing, simple call-and-recall, and word processing. However, there was considerable variation in the effectiveness with which the computers were used. For example, most of the high-use practices had ceased to pull notes when using the computer to issue repeat prescriptions. This enabled substantial time saving. By contrast, most of the other computer practices continued to pull notes, and many of these merely used the computer as a printer, checking eligibility against notes rather than against the computer record.

Thus the effectiveness of computer use appeared to be patchy, and rather disappointing in relation to some of the high expectations reported at the outset of the 'Micros for GPs' scheme. Similarly there were few signs that the computer had been used to generate any substantial income (e.g. through increased items of service payments), nor was there any overall saving in doctors' or staff time. In fact there was a tendency for more extensive computer use to be associated with more employed staff. Moreover, a hope that computer use might reduce prescribing costs through more generic prescribing was not confirmed. Although several practices used the computer to support a generic prescribing policy, these practices were largely those that had a commitment to generic prescribing prior to computerisation.

Despite the limited achievements with the computer in terms of the assessed effects, the vast majority of users (doctors and staff) were enthusiastic about the computer in the practice, and the doctors were generally more positive than the staff. Over 70 per cent of doctors saw the computer as providing a superior means of carrying out registrations, repeat prescribing and preventive procedures. Very few wished to revert to manual procedures.

The study identified a number of factors which influenced the effectiveness of computer use. An important factor that distinguished doctors in the high-use practices from the others was their level of commitment to developing the organisation and its services. Practices that made little effective use of their computer may have started with enthusiastic GPs, but in the event they tended to leave the computer to their staff and did not see the need for their active involvement in the management of the process. However, to ensure that desired outcomes are achieved requires the application of particular managerial skills. The practice needs to determine the action required to implement the computer project effectively. It needs to plan, co-ordinate and review these actions.

The doctors also needed to agree standards for the categorisation of information, and procedures for systematically and reliably collecting and updating it. This was particularly difficult in some practices because GPs traditionally tend to work independently from one another, and rarely need to agree details of procedure. It was not uncommon for find doctors failing to adhere to previously agreed procedures. This could create serious problems in an information system shared among the whole partnership.

Poor design of the computer systems could also be an inhibiting factor. The study found that some systems were slow, had poorly designed preventive facilities, inadequate report generating functions, and generally were not very 'user-friendly'. However, for any particular type of system there was a range in the effectiveness with which it was used, and the Report[3] concluded: 'We do not regard their design as the major impediment to development, although at times inadequate features can slow down progress' (p. 43).

The computer in the consultation

We have also been involved in some studies of computer use during consultations. We have looked at how a group of GPs used a system that had computer-based medical notes and patient management protocols, and, in a separate study, how some hospital doctors and some GPs used a computerised diagnostic aid. Formalised diagnostic aids are not common in general practice, although the adoption of protocols for the management of chronic conditions has become more feasible with the use of computers.

Our main focus has been on the impact of the computer on the consultation process and its acceptability to doctor and patient. This research was originally stimulated by a concern expressed in a report of the RCGP Computer Working Party,[5] which stated: 'We have an important reservation about this development. We do not know whether direct input into the computer during the consultation will have an effect on doctor/patient communication.'

To study the impact on the consultation we have video-recorded about 1000 consultations, some with and some without computer use for comparison. Two systems have been assessed in this way. The first was a decision aid for the diagnosis of patients presenting with dyspepsia,[6] and the other was the IBM Sheffield Primary Care System, a comprehensive experimental general practice system (see ref. 7 for an overview of the system and its evaluation). In this section space permits only a brief summary of the main results obtained. References to full reports are provided for the interested reader to pursue.

In both the studies there was considerable variation in the way doctors chose to use the computer. 'Minimal' users tried to 'protect' the patient from direct exposure to the computer. Some did this most of the time, others only when they felt they had a sensitive case which demanded that they devote their full attention to the patient. Some of the doctors used the computer extensively whilst the patient was present (the 'conversational' strategy), and involved the patient in the process by letting them look at the screen, or by talking or making a joke about the computer.

The minimal strategy had the advantage for the doctors of not having to share their attention between patient and computer — two very different communication processes which some of the doctors reported were difficult to mix. This was partly due to the design of the system. In the study of the dyspepsia diagnostic aid we were able to propose some redesign criteria to reduce this difficulty.[8] The disadvantage of the minimal strategy was that the doctor had to delay entry of symptoms, and that this resulted in less information being entered and with more distortions.[9]

In both studies it was found that more time was spent using the computer than had previously been devoted to manual notes. This did, of course, influence the doctors' perceptions of the computer and their commitment to using it.

The computer can provide structure to the consultation. This is particularly the case where the computer requests specific symptom information. Use of the dyspepsia system, for example, resulted in all the users collecting more 'computer-relevant' information from the patients. When a computer-based hypertension protocol was used, users focused on 'protocol symptoms' but were *less* concerned with topics that were not part of the protocol.[10]

For entering clinical information a computer system can be designed to permit the use of either 'free text', for example a description of the patient's symptoms in the doctor's own words, or entries from a predetermined and limited set of categories, for example that a particular symptom is present or absent. The IBM Sheffield Primary Care System used the former method for entry of encounter notes. Our observations of its use suggest that there was considerable variation in the way that doctors made entries, that they were discouraged from providing extensive information because of their lack of typing skill, and that the information was therefore sparse, variable and extremely difficult to use for any analyses which required the aggregation of data.[11,12]

The dyspepsia system used predefined symptom categories. We found that data entry was much more complete, though the doctors began to formulate questions to the patient so as to elicit answers that readily fitted into the categories required. Also the computer seemed to encourage the doctors to provide information on symptoms which they had not directly elicited from the patient, but had probably been inferred from other information provided. The doctors also appeared to have difficulties adopting the *terminology* which had been used to predefine the categories. They tended to use their own definitions, resulting in computer entries which did not correspond with what 'should' have been entered using the 'correct' definition of symptoms.[9] Record systems based on predefined categories require that users have sufficient training so that they are familiar with symptom definitions.

The use of a computer structures certain aspects of the consultation. That is not to say, of course, that the doctor is totally constrained. A well-designed system will give the user considerable flexibility and freedom to choose how and when to use it. Nevertheless, it is through having a structure that benefits are made possible. For example, benefits derive through the uniformity and consistency that a structure imposes on data collection, or the prompts and reminders of a management protocol impose on a consultation. However, to enable the potential benefits to be realised the system must have a structure that is appropriate and acceptable to the doctor.

SOME STRATEGIC DEVELOPMENTS IN GENERAL PRACTICE COMPUTING

It is important to place these lessons learned into a wider context. They can then be understood in relation to experiences with the development of information technology (IT) applications in other areas. In this section we will attempt to analyse why GP computing has not as yet fulfilled some of the early high expectations, and also examine the possible consequences of further developments in GP computing.

Table 20.1 lists four 'myths' which appear to have been common expectations of the benefits of GP computing (and may still be for many GPs). Alongside each statement is an explanation, based on research findings, of why it is a myth.

One problem with the development of GP computing, in common with many other IT developments, is that they are led by an initiative to *promote the technology*, rather than to identify a *service need*, and then investigate how the technology may be used as a tool to meet that need. The 'Micros for GPs' scheme was sponsored by the Department of Trade and Industry primarily to promote the British computer industry. In a much wider review of IT developments a recent government-sponsored report[13] has commented:

> In the short term most expectations are for . . . doing what is already done a little better, as when word processors replace typewriters or electronic components electro-mechanical ones. To a large extent this generation of products and services reflects a strong 'technology push' emphasis: user needs have not yet been clearly understood or examined, and so the range of products and services emerging is based mostly on reproducing those already in existence. (p. 49).

Table 20.1: Explanations for 'myths' related to GP computing

Myth	Finding/Explanation
1. IT will increase the efficiency of the practice, and therefore:	This does not happen in most practices during the first two years:
(a) After some teething troubles, due mainly to 'user-attitudes', the practice will run more smoothly.	(a) The introduction of IT is like using a dentist's disclosing tablet. It *reveals* inffective organization which is dormant. In itself it is not a cure.
(b) Less people will be needed to do the same work once IT is installed.	(b) *More* work, not less, is required if the computer is to be used effectively. This is partly because the computer does not necessarily save time on the old tasks, and partly because it provides new opportunities which require staff and doctor time.
2. Once a system has been chosen and bought most GPs do not need to involve themselves in the implementation and use of 'administrative' systems. This is a job for the office staff. The GP's work will not be affected in any significant way.	Effective computer use, even for administrative systems, requires commitment and active involvement from all the GPs as part of a co-ordinated information management strategy.
3. If consulting room systems are used, they will improve information handling, but will not impose any constraints on the way the GPs work.	Consulting room systems can improve information handling, but are likely to *increase* the time spent processing information. They will impose a structure on the GPs' way of working. Effective use *requires* adherence to this structure.
4. The technology is *the* problem. And therefore all will be well when the next generation of systems arrive.	Although there is clearly room for improvement, with both software and hardware, the way that systems are implemented and used is of key importance.

Outlined below are seven processes which are particularly relevant in the development of information technology. The concepts underlying these processes derive from a range of studies of information technology and organisational change. However, they help one to understand some of the current findings in general practice, and to anticipate how things may develop in the future.

1. Information management

In a 'business' organisation there will be established routines for processing information (orders, invoices, stock levels, customer accounts, etc.), and the viability of the enterprise *depends* on them being managed effectively. However, at the moment general practice is not operationally or financially dependent on systematic procedures for the processing of clinical information. Thus in most practices there are few such systematic processes. For example, prior to computerisation the procedures of data definition, systematic collection and analysis rarely exist. Thus when a computer is introduced as an aid to information management, these *additional* tasks must be carried out. Whereas in a business organisation a computer can help streamline these tasks, in general practice it leads to their creation. It is fairly common, also, for manual procedures that do exist to be retained, for example age–sex registers or repeat prescribing cards. This explains why computerisation can lead to *more work*. It is part of the process of creating effective information management.

2. Augmentation of service provision

Computerisation can also lead to service innovations. With the availability of a computer, for example, practices set up more preventive programmes. Thus the computer is a catalyst to new activities, but these, of course, entail *extra work* for the practice and its staff. Any benefits in terms of a reduction in acute consultations would only show up in the longer term, if at all.

3. Standardisation of information processing

Our studies, summarised in the previous section, have found that using a computer in the consultation necessarily leads to increased standardisation of clinical information, to a tendency to focus in a consultation on topics covered by the computer, and in some circumstances to a structuring of the consultation process itself. This standardisation can be *beneficial* to clinical decision-making, but it must also be recognised as a *constraint* on the doctor, who must be aware of the circumstances in which the predetermined structure becomes *inappropriate*.[14]

4. Substitution of manual processes

In industrial and office settings it is common to use information technology to substitute for existing manual activities or functions. This usually happens in two stages: *rationalisation* followed by *automation*. The development of computer services in the clearing banks over the past 20 years demonstrates this. Firstly, the main customer transactions (withdrawing and paying in) were formalised and standardised (for example, through the use of paying-in slips), and at the same time other customer services, which were hard to formalise, were separated off. This simplified the task for counter clerks, who therefore required less training. The next stage was to automate the formalised processes. Thus most banks now have auto-tills to substitute for counter clerks in the main transactions.

It is interesting to speculate whether similar processes will occur in general practice. A potential candidate for the two-stage substitution process is the consultation itself. It seems extremely unlikely that all consultations could be formalised, so the first step in the rationalisation process would need to be a separation of tasks into those that could be formalised and those that would be too difficult. The former might include consultations for certain chronic illnesses. In fact this formalisation has already begun with the development of patient management protocols. Through these it is possible to introduce another type of substitution — that of less highly trained paramedical staff. The development of full automation would require computer systems with which patients interacted directly. These would need to incorporate safeguards, such as an indication to the patient of the occasions when it was necessary to consult a doctor.

We are not arguing that these developments will necessarily happen, nor that they are desirable. But we are suggesting that developments that have taken place in other areas could have direct parallels in health care.

5. Enabling or disabling technologies?

One of the reported benefits of computers in general practice is that, used effectively, they allow GPs to feel more in control of their practice — to have a better understanding of what is going on, to focus their efforts with greater confidence and therefore to derive more job satisfaction. In contrast, the substitution process of formalisation and automation, described above, would probably leave health care workers with a sense of having less personal control over their day-to-day work. The outcome which occurs in practice will depend on *the way* that the technology is developed and applied.

The trend towards more preventive programmes also has implications for the control that patients have over their health care. The more pro-active that GPs become in initiating contacts with patients, for example call-and-recall, the less need there will be for patients to take the initiative. Arguably, at the moment the 'decision to consult' is the most active step that patients take in their health care; once in the consulting room their role becomes relatively passive. This issue is considered in more depth in Fitter,[15] and is also discussed by Stott in Chapter 18 of this book. Again, depending on the way that it is developed, the technology could be enabling or disabling for patients.

6. Managerial control of general practice

GPs have a dual role in their practice. They are both practitioners and owners/managers of a business. Information systems can be used to support both roles. Clinical aids fit into the practitioner role. The development of better management information systems can support the role of the GP as manager. This can include monitoring of clinical and administrative processes and assessment of individual or practice performance. Such information can be used to improve practice management and resource planning.

Recently there has been increased interest in audit in general practice, in particular by the Royal College of General Practitioners.[16] The favoured form is peer-group review,[17] and a recent study using a computer to audit the activities of a partnership is reported by Fitter, Evans and Garber.[18] However, there may be pressures in the future to make health and performance data available outside the practice — either to the DHSS as paymasters, or to patients as clients. It is interesting to observe that the clearing banks are now *required* by law to make summary statistics regularly available to the government. It would have been *impossible* in practice to provide them prior to computerisation. Thus the discerning GP might see the computer in general practice either as a 'combine harvester' efficiently reaping an immense volume of data for the benefit of the practice, or alternatively as a 'Trojan horse' opening up general practice to outside scrutiny.

7. Integration of primary health care

Because of its independent status general practice is not fully integrated into the primary health care service. Community health services operate separately and with their own information systems. It will be dysfunctional and detrimental to patients if general practice and community services continue to develop their systems separately, and the recent report from the Social Services Committee[19] recommends that: 'the Government take urgent steps to enable DHAs and FPCs to share information on the health and health needs of their area, including information held on computer databases'.

The problems of integration are, in the main, not technical. The difficulties of agreeing a common framework have been identified in an editorial of the Newsletter of the Primary Care Specialist Group of the British Computer Society in July 1986 as being essentially political: 'The basis for their disagreement was not on clinical, logistical or data accuracy grounds but what appeared to be a generally held view that "he who holds the index [of patients] has all power"' (p. 2). Information technology could also prove useful for integrating general practice into hospital services, for example linking to pathology laboratories for test results, and directly to wards to communicate details on the discharge of patients. Such developments are beginning to take place,[20] but there is much still to be done.

THE ROLE OF THE GENERAL PRACTITIONER: TWO SCENARIOS

From the array of issues concerning the development of general practice computing identified above, we wish to draw out one theme which cuts across several issues, and is central to the future of general practice. How will the role of the general practitioner develop? Because we believe it must. Outlined below are two contrasting scenarios with some possible associated implications.

Scenario 1: The GP as manager

There is a growing pressure that GPs should see themselves more as businessmen and women, running an efficient and profitable organisation. This view has been combined with another trend — a desire to make general practice more responsive to consumers — in the proposal outlined in the recent Government Green Paper[21] that 'health shops' be established. The arguments underlying this have been most clearly stated by Alan Maynard: 'My preference is for capitalism and experimentation with the development of market mechanisms in the NHS. To ensure GPs can compete with each other for customers some radical changes are needed. (*Pulse*, 15 October 1986, p. 30).

The aim is to increase the accountability of GPs, to ensure 'value for money' and to do it through market mechanisms. Possible consequences of this scenario are the direct charging of patients for services received, particularly for preventive services, as has been proposed by the BMA. Another consequence might be to accelerate the development of IT for *substitution* as described in process 4 above, i.e. that jobs now done by people will be taken over by computer or by paramedical staff instead of doctors. Decision aids for patients about whether to consult, or advice on minor illness in telephone consultations, are examples where substitution would 'free' the doctor's time for other activities, such as management of the business.

Scenario 2: The GP as practitioner

The traditional role of the GP is as practitioner, and as the carer and the main point of contact for patients. There are some who see this still as the vital role, and who also see IT as an opportunity to reestablish it in practice, having managed to pass off as many of the administrative and management responsibilities as possible. For example, in a discussion of the use of IT in the community health services (CHIP), Geoffrey Clayton[22] has concluded:

> I would say three cheers for CHIPs as I understand it if it means the removal of a considerable administrative burden from general practice leaving us with the role for which we thought we had been trained. Namely face to face contact in the consultation, a long term friendly relationship with our patients and intercessor on their behalf with the rest of the health industry (p. 32).

This view is in sharp contrast to the developing role of the GP as manager. It will appeal to a substantial number of GPs who have neither the inclination, nor the necessary skills, to act as managers.

It will be difficult for GPs to avoid an increase in the management role if general practice continues to be organised as it is now, and the trend towards larger organisational units and a wider range of services continues, as seems likely. Thus in this alternative scenario the future GP will work as a *practitioner* in a primary care team, alongside other health care professionals, each with their own specific role. The management of such a unit would probably require the services of a general manager/administrator. One organisational form has been proposed in the Cumberlege Report,[23] in which a neighbourhood centre would provide primary care services to a local population. This could enable information systems to be used to assess and plan resource requirements in a flexible way to meet local needs, and would depend on 'health care associations' rather than market mechanisms as the means of providing accountability to patients.

Both of these scenarios anticipate that GPs will become more accountable to their client group, but with very different mechanisms for doing so. Which scenario will provide a better service to patients and better value for money?

Further evaluations will be necessary, and not just on technical aspects. It is important that future evaluations assess developments against health care objectives, including improvements in health outcomes, and also in terms of economic objectives (organisational effectiveness and cost) and personal objectives (job quality and service quality).

These evaluations could take the form of pilot projects assessing alternative organisational forms, for example as outlined in the two scenarios above, and of other variants based upon them. Now is the time to experiment, assess and choose. Otherwise general practitioners will find themselves swept through the crossroads without having made a decision on which way they want to go.

ACKNOWLEDGEMENTS

We gratefully acknowledge financial support from the Department of Health and Social Security, and from the IBM UK Scientific Centre, for the research described in the chapter. We also thank Joan Harrison and Guy Herzmark for helpful comments on an earlier draft.

REFERENCES

1. Friedson, E. (1970) *The profession of medicine*. Harper & Row, New York
2. Fitter, M.J. (1987) The development and use of information technology in health care. In: Blackler, F. and Oborne, D. (eds), *Information technology and people: designing for the future*. British Psychological Society, Leicester
3. DHSS (1985) *General practice computing, evaluation of the Micros for GPs' scheme: final report*. HMSO, London
4. DHSS (1986) *A prescription for change: a report on the longer term use and development of computers in general practice*. HMSO, London
5. RCGP Computer Working Party (1980) *Computers in primary care*. Occasional Paper 13. Royal College of General Practitioners, London
6. Barber, D.C. and Fox, J. (1981) First aid: a design philosophy and program for on-line symptom processing. *International Journal of Bio Medical Computing*, 12, 249–65
7. Fitter, M.J., Brownbridge, G., Garber, J.R. and Herzmark, G.A. (1985) A human factors evaluation of the IBM Sheffield Primary Care system. In: Shackel, B. (ed), *Human–computer interaction — INTERACT '84*. Elsevier Science Publishers, North Holland
8. Fitter, M.J. and Cruickshank, P.J. (1982) The computer in the consulting room: a psychological framework. *Behaviour and Information Technology*, 1, 81–92
9. Brownbridge, G., Fitter, M.J. and Sime, M. (1984). The doctor's use of a computer in the consulting room: an analysis. *International Journal of Man–Machine Studies*, 21, 65–90
10. Brownbridge, G., Evans, A., Fitter, M. and Platts, M. (1986) An interactive computerized protocol for the management of hypertension: Effects on the General Practitioner's clinical behaviour. *Journal of the Royal College of General Practitioners*, 36, 198–202
11. Herzmark, G.A., Brownbridge, G., Fitter, M. and Evans, A. (1984). Consultation use of a computer by General Practitioners. *Journal of the Royal College of General Practitioners*, 34, 649–54
12. Evans, A. and Brownbridge, G. (1985). Computer use within the consultation: the Sheffield experience. In: Sheldon, M. and Stoddart, M. (eds), *Trends in general practice computing*. Royal College of General Practitioners, London
13. Long-term Perspectives Group of Information Technology EDC (1986) *IT Futures: what current forecasting literature says about the social impact of information technology*. National Economic Development Corporation, London
14. Fitter, M.J. (1985) A discussion on aids to decision-making in the consultation. In: Sheldon, M., Brooke, J. and Rector, A. (eds), *Decision-making in general practice*. Macmillan, Basingstoke
15. Fitter, M.J. (1986) Evaluation of computers in primary health care: the effect on doctor–patient communication. In: Peterson, H.E. and Schneider, W. (eds), *Human–computer communications in health care*. Elsevier Science Publishers, North Holland
16. RCGP (1985) *Quality of general practice: policy statement 2*. Royal

College of General Practitioners, London

17. Reilly, R.M. and Patten, M.P. (1978) An audit of prescribing by peer review. *Journal of the Royal College of General Practitioners*, 28, 525-30

18. Fitter, M.J., Evans, A.R. and Garber, J.R. (1985). Computers and audit. *Journal of the Royal College of General Practitioners*, 35, 522-4

19. Social Services Committee (1987) *Primary health care*, Volume 1 (First Report, Session 1986-7). HMSO, London

20. Hewett, D.J. and Thurston, F. (1987) Building the network backwards. Paper presented to Current Perspectives in Healthcare Computing Conference, Cardiff

21. Government 'Green Paper' (1986) *Primary health care: an agenda for discussion.* HMSO, London

22. Clayton, G. (1987) The information needs of general practice. *Newsletter of the Primary Care Specialist Group of the British Computer Society*, 4(5), 27-32

23. Cumberlege Report (1986). *Neighbourhood Nursing – A Focus for Care: Report of the Community Nursing Review.* HMSO, London

21

The Final Account

Richard Turner

INTRODUCTION

At the height of the Second World War the coalition government thought it was important to start planning for postwar Britain. Sir William Beveridge was commissioned to produce the famous report on social and allied services (Cmd. 6404) which contained his suggestions for fighting the 'five giant evils' of want, disease, ignorance, squalor and idleness in the postwar world.[1] The 1948 National Health Service Act gave responsibility for administering the Health Service to the Ministry of Health, together with responsibility for supervising non-medical provision for the elderly and handicapped by local authorities.

However, the Home Office was given responsibility for looking after neglected children, the Ministry of Education for School Health, the Ministry of Labour for Occupational Health and the Ministry of National Insurance for running the universal National Insurance Scheme for Social Security.

In 1971 it was recognised that the evils still remained. All personal social services were brought together under the umbrella of the Department of Health and Social Security in an attempt to unify them. A single minister was given charge over the whole health and welfare field, and it was hoped that the separate services would henceforth co-operate to provide care to those who needed it as, where, when and how it could be provided most economically.

Unfortunately the task proved too great, and the 'DH' and 'SS' remained virtually independent of one another.

As a result the hospital services currently have to be planned in ignorance of the true incidence or prevalence of disease in the community. Providers of primary care have to cope without being able to arrange non-emergency hospital care as and when their patients require it; and the Social Services cannot arrange for medical treatment even when they know that a minor operation might save a considerable sum in benefit payments to the family.

In 1974, 1982 and 1984 successive reorganisations of the NHS each tried to take account of these problems as far as they related to the health service, and the general managers of the current era have been specifically charged with moving care into the community wherever possible.

However, it can be argued that until communications between the hospital and the community services are improved, the burden of actually communicating will defeat the objective of inducing them to co-operate more closely. The question must therefore be: are there any insurmountable objections to improving communications?

The thesis of this chapter is that they will be improved much sooner than most people would expect, and that this will have a considerable impact on the way in which primary care services operate.

A JOURNAL OF CURRENT EVENTS

Over the past ten years the need for computers on a large scale in the health service has been increasingly recognised by epidemiologists and research workers, but until recently there seemed no hope of information services being thought to be of sufficient importance to justify the very considerable expenditure which was obviously going to be required.

Within a period of three years, however, an extraordinary set of events has occurred which has completely altered the outlook, and opportunities are now opening up which might otherwise have taken a lifetime.

The first 'event' was the publication of the Korner reports. For the first time agreement was reached between all authorities that a minimum amount of standard data relating to every patient and every aspect of NHS care (with a few important exceptions) should be collected on a regular basis.

Every Region is now committed to collect the minimum data sets in their entirety by 1 April 1988. Many have employed management consultants to assist with the production of Region-wide information and computing strategies based on the Korner requirements, and the scale of expenditure expected over the next eight to ten years ranges from £24m to £75m per Region.

The next event was the acceptance by the government of the Griffiths recommendations on the reorganisation of management arrangements within the Hospital and Community Health Services — the HCHS as the NHS is now referred to in all official publications.[2]

Implementation of these proposals was presented publicly as a relatively minor administrative rearrangement, but it has in fact led to a complete change in organisation of the service, and to a reinterpretation of the role of HCHS Authorities.

At first sight the new role looks precisely the same as before, and it can be summarised as 'To make the best use of limited resources to improve the health of the population.' Nothing much new there, one might think. However, the change lies in the emphasis now placed on the words.

Making the 'best' use of resources is seen as being the responsibility of each HCHS level of Authority through its general manager. Instead of DHAs being responsible for making up their own minds on which services should have priority, the current theme is 'accountability downwards, responsibility upwards'. The system of financial rewards to managers is in fact to depend on their ability to bring about changes specified by the Department of Health and implemented by the new management units (co-ordinated and monitored by DHAs and RHAs respectively).

From an information point of view this means that, both nationally and locally, managers must have accurate and up-to-date information relating to the set objectives and to all the circumstances which may affect their achievement. The objectives themselves will be related to the level of service provided to patients, and it will no longer be sufficient for authorities to demonstrate that so many beds or staff per 1000 population have been provided. The requirement, as in industry, will be to assess the use made of assets such as buildings, staff and equipment, and to make changes where these are not being deployed effectively.

The fact that resources are now 'limited' means that new developments must be funded by closing down other services which are no longer 'required'. This can be expected to lead to a new demand for more accurate information as different contenders for expenditure argue their case.

Part of 'Improving the health of the population' will relate to prevention (improving the proportions of population immunised or screened, as well as reducing morbidity and mortality), and if the prescribed levels are not achieved, HCHS managers will have to pay more attention to the organisation and evaluation of these services throughout the District. They will have to liaise with independent contractors and decide for themselves how such services can best be provided on a district-by-district basis. The same will apply to hospital services.

Altering the responsibilities of Health Authorities from merely providing adequate facilities for health care to ensuring that they are used effectively means that the quantity, quality and level of detail of data to be collected, processed, analysed and interpreted will have to be increased out of all proportion to that currently handled.

However, the new management will not be able to manage without it, and it is this which has led to actual expenditure on information services on an unprecedented scale. As mentioned above, there is no Region in the country which will not have spent literally millions of pounds on computers to collect and process the Korner data sets by 1 April 1988.

The last 'extraordinary event' relates to the development of an NHS Data Model.

Given that data will be collected mainly as a by-product of day-to-day operational use of the computers, the problem which arises is how to store and organise it all in such a way that both those who provided it, and the managers who are responsible for running the service, can make use of it.

The Korner committee's recommendations did include standard definitions of terms, which are essential if comparable statistics are to be obtained from different hospitals or DHAs, but they said nothing about how the vast amount of raw data should be collected or stored in such a way that it can be aggregated in different ways for different purposes.

The problem can be illustrated by considering the simple card index in general practice. Everyone knows that if there is requirement to look out all the patients with asthma one day, and all the patients who have had a recent cervical smear the next, then two separate card indexes will be needed, and for patients with asthma who also need a cervical smear, the patient identification details will have to be duplicated on each.

Computers can use any field in the patient record as a basis for selecting records (i.e. as a 'key'), but obviously they cannot use information which is not recorded at all. If the practice wishes to analyse which partners are doing most home visits, for example, then both the fact that the patient was seen at home and the identification of the doctor doing the visit must be recorded on the relevant patient record on each occasion.

If the frequency of home visits within a given DHA, rather than within a single practice, is to be analysed (i.e. leaving out those patients on any doctor's list which live in another DHA) then a code identifying the DHA will also have to be added. So far, three extra items have been added to the patient record. If there is then a requirement to look at home visiting by senior as opposed to junior partners, or by male as opposed to female doctors, or by rich and poor areas of town rather than by DHA, then either the enquirer will have to remember which doctor and address falls into which category or yet further items of data will have to be added to the patient record to enable them to be sorted into the appropriate groups.

THE DATA MODEL

The principle of the data model is to keep all records in a hierarchical set of files, and to provide links between these, rather than attempt to keep a single large patient file and put all these extra items and codes on to every patient record.

To take the example given above, the set of linked files (which could just be card indexes if no computers exist) would include the following:

(A) practices in the district
(B) doctors in each practice
(C) patients registered with each doctor
(D) addresses classified by 'social class' of area
(E) appointment file for each doctor (see Figure 21.1)

Every record in every file has a link number showing which record in the file it relates to. Thus a lot of patients in the 'patient' file would have the same link number to a single record in the 'doctor' file, because they were all registered with the same doctor. This is known as a 'one-to-many' relationship.

Given a computer program which is designed to work with linked files, each of the queries in the above example relating to home visiting patterns can be answered *without* all the information about the doctor having to be duplicated on the records of each of his patients.

Figure 21.1

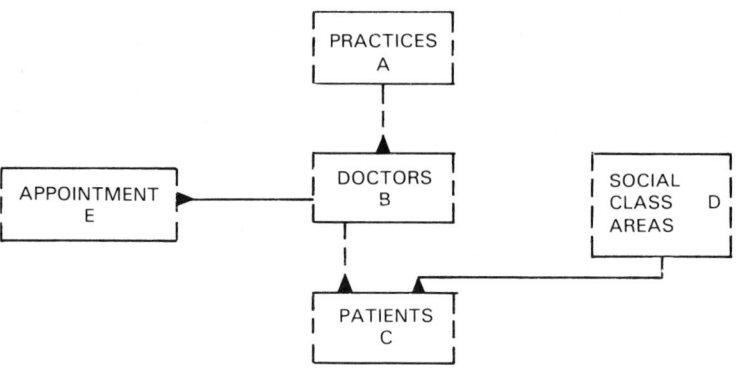

To look at another aspect, it might be of interest to see if the younger patients always chose the younger doctors. With a single 'flat' patient file one cannot tabulate the ages of doctors in a practice against the ages of their patients (in the above example) unless the age of the doctor is recorded on *every patient record*. With a system of linked files the age of the doctors has only to be recorded on the records in the 'doctor' file, i.e. on six records for a six-doctor practice.

With linked files it is interesting to note that most of the above enquiries can be answered even if they were not envisaged when the filing systems were first established.

This is in marked contrast to the situation when purely patient-based computer files or card indexes are used, since few enquirers could be bothered to go right through the patient file adding the appropriate codes.

When something extra is required, another link file can just be added. In the above example the requirement to analyse numbers of patients in each social class area may not have been thought of originally. With a 'flat' patient file a 'social class' code would have to be inserted next to the address on every patient record. If six people live at the same address the code would have to be added to the record for each one. With a linked-file system an extra file grouping addresses into social class districts can be added to the system, and the enquiry made *via* that, without having to amend every patient record.

The science of converting the notebooks, card indexes, ledgers and files used in the day-to-day running of any practice or hospital into a set of linked files which can be used to answer any query is known as data modelling.

The technique has in fact been used for years in many international corporations, but it is new to the Health Service because it is only really relevant to computerised filing systems, and the NHS has up until now made very little use of computers except for financial purposes. A data base of linked files is known as a relational data base, and the individual files relating to, say, patients, doctors and locations, are known as entities, each of which has various attributes (such as age of doctor or whatever), and relationships (i.e. links) to other files.

A data dictionary is usually created with definitions of all entities, attributes and relationships and, provided this is kept up to date, interrogation programs can be employed which do not have to be rewritten whenever fields are added to or deleted from the individual records in any file.

Furthermore, the system of linking files lends itself ideally to distributed computer systems. As long as each computer can be linked to the others directly or over telephone wires, files can be held on disc anywhere in the network, and accessed by having each computer 'phone' others in sequence down the chain. This solves the necessity for vast amounts of data actually to have to be transported from one computer to another in order that one computer can have access to data held by another.

Programming tools even exist which can take a properly designed data model on one hand, and certain information about how often which files will be accessed by whom, etc., on the other, and produce an entire computer filing system automatically. Such a design will take into account which computer should physically hold what data on its discs according to who in the network requires the most frequent access to it.

An NHS data model covering all aspects of hospital and primary care has been constructed over a period of years, and is now available.[3] It includes as entities and attributes all financial, manpower, activity and patient data normally to be found in the hospital and in community records at the present time. Although it is only a set of diagrams on paper accompanied by a data dictionary, it provides a framework within which individual computer systems running on any hardware can in principle all be linked together. Extra linked files can of course be added, and as time goes by this model will be developed just as a public library can be enlarged by adding books either in that library or by enabling it to locate and call for books from another library.

A District-wide system based on the data model will, however, have certain capabilities which go beyond those of present systems based on flat files.

THE BOOK OF LIFE

Perhaps the most interesting of these is that they can bring together all the details relating to *care* provided to a given patient over any period of time. They are not limited to the finite amount of information which can be stored and processed by any single machine, or by the necessity for all the relevant facts to be collected together in one place and added to the patient record, as current systems are.

Given the expansion capability, linked computer systems can accumulate information about just who did what for which patients over long periods of time, and make it accessible to whoever is authorised to search for information via the network (unlike manual records or single computer systems which can only make information available to those who can travel to the computer centre or get hold of the pieces of paper the record is written on).

The foundations for a 'Book of Life' to be built up for every person in the country are in place now.

To start with, the National Child Health Computer system, now used by over half the Health Authorities in England and Wales, first learns of the existence of a new baby when details from the statutory Birth Notification Form are entered into it. Alternatively, the midwife delivering the baby enters the details into the computer before she leaves the labour ward, and it generates the birth notification form, with copies for the Registrar and the case notes. The computer waits for three months or so until the first immunisation or check-up visit (for babies notified to it as being 'at-risk') is due, when it makes the necessary arrangements and reports on non-attenders. All changes of address and movements of children in and out of districts are reported to the system to ensure that courses of immunisation are completed, and that at-risk children are followed up.

The registration and immunisation modules of this system have now been followed by the pre-school health and school health modules, which arrange screening, follow-up and immunisation appointments until the child leaves school. The system runs on Regional mainframe computers, as do the hospital activity, personnel, payroll and accounting systems in most Regional Health Authorities.

Most districts are also now installing hospital patient administration systems (PAS) which handle all requests for biochemical and other investigations, record drug therapy, arrange operating theatre sessions, etc., and of course they keep records of all this activity as required under the Korner proposals.

At the same time Family Practitioner Committees are becoming computerised, and it has been recognised[4] that there would be potential advantages in linking practice computers to these, and thence to Health Authority machines. FPC patient indexes could in fact be used in place of hospital patient indexes, which would avoid the considerable duplication of effort required to create and maintain duplicate indexes.

GPs could then book outpatient appointments directly from the surgery, and then use their computer systems both to access laboratory reports relating to their patients and to read copies of letters held on hospital computer files, rather than have to *transfer* the said letters to their own computer systems, and waste storage space. All that would be required would be the appropriate links.

A NATIONAL HEALTH SERVICE?

Information on the size and health status of the population is currently collected and published by a whole range of institutions besides those which collect it as a by-product of the processes of health care.

The most important is the Office of Population Censuses and Surveys (OPCS) which collects details of births, marriages, and deaths, and conducts the Decennial National Census, as well as carrying out various national surveys including the General Household Survey.

Given that births are notified both to the NHS and to the Registrar of Births, and that the registrar requires to have confirmation from the midwife that a baby was in fact delivered before he will register it, there would seem to be a good case for the registrar having access to the NHS computer network directly.

In return, it would facilitate studies relating to the incidence and effectiveness of treatment in cancer and other fatal diseases (not to mention the work of hospital and GP record departments) if the NHS network could be notified automatically when the patient dies, and of the cause of death.

Such information is conveyed manually at present, and print-outs from the OPCS computer can be laboriously entered into individual computer systems if it is known which systems have records relating to which patients. From the confidentiality point of view, the direct link would merely be more efficient.

It would also be useful if notifications of infectious disease could be made direct to the immunisation module of the child health system. This would enable statistics to be produced routinely on which courses of immunisation were ineffective (for whatever reason), and provide firm evidence on which communities were falling seriously behind others as far as their state of protection was concerned (again for whatever reason).

Studies of the effect of immunisation on unrelated illnesses such as cancer or rheumatoid arthritis, which may or may not have a direct relationship to immunisation against the common infectious diseases, could also be carried out.

Apart from improving the transfer of information, there are also ways in which primary care services could co-operate more with the hospital services, to their mutual advantage, if communications were improved. The obvious area for consideration is 'care in the community'.

Patients could perhaps be discharged earlier from hospital if the consultant could be sure that services in the community were available to look after them from the date of discharge, or if he could actually enter the required visits and factors which should be checked into the diary of the appropriate member of the primary health care team. In return, GPs should be able to book hospital places directly for their more urgent cases (and this should not only include cases in which life was threatened).

Obviously either opportunity could be abused, and it might be wise to limit it to a given proportion of the total resource available (at least initially). In time, direct communications, together with facilities for on-line confirmation, say at the end of each day, could build up confidence.

Other forms of co-operation could be instituted such as the 'shared care' agreements between consultants and GPs in relation to diabetes which are operated in many districts now. Joint GP/

consultant clinics in the community or in the hospital could be arranged automatically when a GP had a sufficient number of patients to justify them, according to jointly agreed criteria.

Various statistics relating to the HCHS locally could also be produced automatically. General practitioners could keep a check on the adequacy and effectiveness of the hospital services (which would be useful to them and to district managers), and hospitals could monitor which practices referred more cases to hospital than others (which certainly happens in some areas).

There are many opinions, and much grumbling, in many districts now, but often little objective evidence; therefore nothing gets done.

The eventual outcome could be a much more efficient National Health Service, as Beveridge originally envisaged.

The interesting point about all this is that if the practical, economic and other arguments for linkage are as valid as they appear (less duplication of indexes, reliable transmission of cervical cytology and other results to the GP, planning based on accurate assessments of morbidity as recorded by GPs for their own purposes, research into the effect various forms of paramedical or drug or manipulative treatment have on long-term patient health, or on hospital admission patterns) then linked systems are likely to be established. Practical and financial arguments have already proved much more substantial in the eyes of the managers and the treasurers of Health Authorities than the requirements of academics which have been put forward over the years, and we now have tools which can overcome the kind of problems experienced by pioneering projects such as the Oxford Record Linkage Study. There is also the point that computer technology is likely to become more powerful and cheaper the more it becomes commonplace.

For the first time ever, it is likely that we may soon have not only a 'Book of Life' relating to every individual born, but also the basis for establishing a truly integrated service without threatening the independence of GPs.

THE FINAL ACCOUNT

Of course, given a properly constructed system, enquiries can also be made relating to the way in which individual doctors investigate, diagnose, treat, refer and follow up their patients, and to the quantity and variety of work carried out by any individual or unit in the HCHS.

A system has already been developed on a microcomputer and installed in many hospitals which enables the consultant in charge of a department to see how his junior staff investigate particular problems, and whether they reach the correct conclusions more often at the end of their training periods than they did at the start, *and* whether they have in fact obtained as wide an experience of treating different patients as is considered desirable.

Such principles can obviously be extended to take the resources used to manage patients in different centres into account (costed using a link file), and to assess whether the patients treated by one doctor subsequently require much more treatment for the same condition than those treated by another. In the final account, use of resources can be related to the results obtained.

The capabilities of such a system will obviously appear threatening to any doctor who has secret fears about his own capabilities or level of activity (and who doesn't!!?)

Several points relating to these fears can, however, be made. The first is that computers only *monitor* such things — they do not make decisions (except in science-fiction stories). All doctors, of course, have their strengths and weaknesses, and on any scale of ability or industry or whatever, the majority will be found sheltering happily under the dome of the bell-shaped curve beloved of statisticians. The science of measurement will have to become very much more exact before the kind of care which patients really appreciate (and which undoubtedly contributes to therapeutic success) can be accurately assessed and entered as data into computer systems. Doctors *are* accountable to their patients, and managers cannot improve anything by misusing information or by drawing the wrong conclusions, however much data they have available to them.

Of course, there will be a few people in any profession who stand out at each end of the normal distribution. Some should undoubtedly receive merit awards, while others could be offered assistance to alter their ways, rather than be penalised in any way. Even if penalties were appropriate in very extreme cases, it would not be an argument against linked systems, since no profession could argue that a system with such potential benefit to the vast majority of both doctors and patients should be banned because of the fears of a small minority.

Who should be entitled to look at what, and be allowed to draw conclusions under what circumstances, however, needs careful consideration, in case data are erroneously interpreted and decisions are taken on the basis of those data without the doctor ever being aware of why circumstances affecting him have been changed.

The Data Protection Act gives protection to patient records but provides little protection for professionals. A District might (conceivably) conclude that patients in a given practice were not being properly followed up because the doctors there did not enter details of uneventful follow-up visits into the computer. If merit awards to general practitioners were to be introduced and allocated in the same secretive way that they are to hospital doctors, then such GPs may never know why they failed to receive one.

Similarly, an individual GP who takes great care may be criticised for not treating as many patients as his colleagues, and be unable to produce evidence from the computer with which to defend himself, but his patients may do better in ways which are hard to measure.

The only answer to the misuse of data in this sense is for doctors to involve themselves in whatever decision-making processes affect them and their patients, or to join organisations which will look after their interests. As the philosopher Proudhon said, the price of freedom is eternal vigilance. Trying to restrict the introduction of linked systems, or access to the system, by 'legislative' means is likely to be unsuccessful since so many people have a legitimate right to count and measure drug prescriptions, item of service claims, hospital referrals, etc., and all those who spend public money must allow appropriate officials to check that it has been properly spent one way or another.

There is also the point that attempts to prevent the introduction of new technology have almost always been unsuccessful in other walks of life.

General practitioners should instead welcome it, but ensure that it is introduced properly, and look forward to having much better records rather than spend any time worrying about any misuse that those properly authorised to have access to the records might make of them.

REFERENCES

1. Cmnd. 6404 Social Insurance and Allied Services (report by Sir William Beveridge) (1942)
2. Great Britain, Department of Health and Social Security (1983) NHS Management Inquiry. (Leader of inquiry: Sir Roy Griffiths). DHSS, London

3. The National Health Service Data Model — Version 1, Volume 1 (Management Summary). NHS Corporate Data Administration, 19 Calthorpe Road, Birmingham B15 1RP

4. Fitter, M.J., Garger, J.R., Herzmark, G.A., Robinson, D. and Jones, R.V.H. (1986) *A Prescription for Change*. HMSO, London

Conclusion: The Way Ahead?

Bob Jones and Richard Westcott

Throughout the first Part of this book the slow struggle to establish a core of health information is painstakingly described. Over nearly two centuries it has been a long march. The impression left by the authors in this and in the second Part is tinged with their impatience and frustration at what still needs to be done. Moreover, as described in Part 3, computers and other electronic technology are not yet being used to fill gaps between present practice and expectations.

In Part 4 the tempo changes. Presented in an unemotional matter-of-fact way, based on their own knowledge and experience, the authors present a compelling vision of the future which will surprise and shock most practitioners. For some the temptation may be to close their eyes and try hard to believe it will never happen. Earlier chapters show that doctors have a long track record of denying information and resisting such changes as may be seen to diminish their status. However, if these changes do occur, and we have little doubt that they will, then patients and the public will have access to information about general health matters and about their own health problems on a scale greater than ever before. The present balance between professionals and patients will change dramatically. The challenges posed to general practitioners by this situation are spelt out in the five final chapters.

Metcalfe presents computers as meta-technology, comparable to the invention of the wheel, as significant and as inevitable. In their separate approaches the others clearly agree with this view.

Johnson, after demonstrating the impossibility of scanning the vast amount of information in computer data bases quickly enough to be of practical use, concludes that digitisation of information is the only answer. His challenge is for the profession to learn a new language, to learn to write in numbers.

CONCLUSION: THE WAY AHEAD?

Metcalfe, Stott, Fitter and Garber are each concerned with aspects of the relationship between doctor, patient and computer.

Pursuing his explicit challenge for family doctors to accept computerisation Metcalfe follows this up by challenging us to accept a computer into the consultation, to remodel the consultation around the computer.

For Stott the information stored about patients on practice computers both clarifies and confuses. The impact of computers on primary care is for better *and* for worse. He quotes the example of a patient for whom a summary of problems and risk factors is misleading; it hides more about the person than it reveals. His challenge, especially to those he calls 'black-and-white thinkers', is to accept the tensions arising from such paradoxes as constructive. Technology should serve rather than drive clinical practice.

Fitter and Garber foresee the computer forcing family doctors to decide whether they are primarily personal doctors or managers. They point out that in industrial and office settings the introduction of information technology commonly leads to rationalisation followed by automation of services. The substitution of auto-tills for counter clerks in banks is a prime example. With these precedents and the current emphasis on practice management their challenge to the profession is to what extent the computer will substitute for the family doctor, with the doctor moving further towards management to the exclusion of personal contact.

Finally Turner, from his position outside general practice, has a wider perspective, as he views the major changes which are occurring in information handling throughout the National Health Service in the UK. As independent contractors general practitioners have been largely unconcerned with this revolution, which involves definition of a basic data set for every person in the country. He describes how linked files will enable analyses to be made of the use of resources and of performance indicators for hospitals, practices and clinicians. Unless general practitioners take part in planning this revolution they will be unable to influence the direction it takes. His challenge to the profession is to participate.

We ourselves have no answers to these challenges. However, in common with our authors we are convinced that major changes will occur within a short time. We fear they will find general practice unprepared.

We invite our profession to discuss the issues which have been presented, to take up these challenges and to decide upon courses of action so that challenge may be turned from threat to opportunity.

Index

A4 record 5, 6, 11
advertising doctors 44
AIDS, Government publicity 56
Alma Ata, Declaration of 84
Annual, The Medical 26
appointments
    and availability 190
    books 187
Arthur Andersen Report 77
artificial intelligence 157–9
Authorities,
    District Health 22, 67, 71, 272
    Health Education *see* Health Education Council

BACUP 54, 82
Book of Life 277
British Medical Journal 26, 28, 33
broadcasting *see* radio, television etc.
Bulletin, Drugs and Therapeutics 36

cable text 215
Campaign for Plain English 47
card
    background data 9
    co-operation 12, 13, 155, 237
    repeat prescription 12, 19
    'smart' 75, 153, 250
    summary 5, 12
Ceefax 108, 213
Census, National 22
Central Office of Information 111
cervical cytology 19, 21, 67
Charter (General Practice Charter) 1965 17, 19, 181
closed user groups 214
codes, computers need 241–51
Cohen
    1950 BMA Committee 27

1964 Report 54
College of Health 83
Collings Report 1950 5
Community Health Councils 45
computers
    acute abdominal pain 139–42
    analysis of records 98
    appointment systems 100
    assisted learning 104, 105, 106, 208–10, 216
    audit 99, 264
    bibliography 101
    billing 89
    codes 241–51
    cost 238–40
    development 223, 238
    diagnosis 131–47
    drug information for doctors 152
    drug information for patients 204
    ethical questions 144–6
    'free' 67
    functions in primary health care 232, 256
    graphics 218–19
    health self-assessment 205, 216, 217
    history taking 104, 205–7, 249
    home 106, 224
    in the consultation 227, 258
    language 244, 259, *see also* Medol, digitisation
    linked files, 18, 230, 274, 278
    myths 261
    out patient appointment booking 194
    paradoxical 233
    patient call and recall 91, 188
    patient information 197–211
    patient registration 91

prescribing 93, 98, 152, 190
preventive procedures 91, 188, *see also* preventive work
research 102
routine recording 99
staff employment 257
strategic developments 260
confidentiality 13, 46, 73, 154, 237
consultation time 104
consumerism 181
Consumers' Association 55
contract of care with individual patient 228
Cormack, study on records 1970 7, 11
Cumberlege Report 1986 267

data base 8, 11, 121
    depersonalising influence of 235
    dictionary 276
    drug 124
    geographic 22, 62
    local 124
    reference 123
    relational 244, 276
    source 123
    structures 243
data modelling 276
data pollution 241
Data Protection Act 74, 282
data, sale of prescribing data 67
Day Book 3
DHSS 107
diabetes 155, 156, 189, 208
digitisation 244–51
Directory, Medical Research 123
Doctor 34

education, postgraduate 27
electronic mail 230
Embase 123

FAMLI 29, 31
flags, 19, 149, 150
floppy disc 121
flow sheet 12, 151

FPC
    computers 67, 278
    helping GPs give information 48
    information to GPs 21
    lists of local GPs 44
    patient turnover 192

General Medical Council, advertising 44
General Practitioner 34
Glasgow dyspepsia system 136
Good Practice Allowance 181
G-Pass software 67, 73
graphics, computer generated 217
Griffiths, recommendations on reorganisation 1983 272

Health Risk Appraisal program 205
health care paradox 234
health education 212–19
Health Education Council 41, 43, 54, 82, 107, 108, 111, 214
health net 154
Health Trends 36
holism 61
hospitals
    bed occupancy 191
    outpatient waiting times 22, 155, 187, 194
    referral rates 193

independent contractor status 253, 265
index, disease 72, 189 *see also* registers, E-Book
Index Medicus 30, 123 *see also* Medline
interactive video 218
item of service payments 21, 181

Jarman Index 71, 194
Joint Committee for Postgraduate Training 10

INDEX

Korner reports 271–3

Lancet 26, 28
leaflets for patients 41, 43, 46, 50, 80, 101, 198
Lloyd George 3
 envelope 63, 151
Local Medical Committees 1971 resolution on A4 6
Loudon
 A4 records 6
 first appearance title 'GP' 25

Mackenzie *Principles of Diagnosis and Treatment in Heart Affections* 1916 26
mandates 183
Martindale-on-Line 74, 123, 244–51
Meditel 107, 123
Medline 101, 123, *see also Index Medicus*
Medol 244
'micros for GPs' scheme 19, 255
MIMS 35
monopoly of professions 46, 50, 53

National Child Health computer system 277
National Consumer Council 45
National Health Service
 its introduction 4, 17
 reorganisations 271
National Health Service Act 1948 270
National Insurance Act 1911 3, 17
Nightingale, Florence 51
numbers, writing in 246–51

Office of Population Censuses and Surveys 278
Oracle, 108, 213
Oxford System of Medicine 126, 159–78
Oxford Textbook of Medicine 171

paradox, the law of 231
patient
 administration systems 278
 autonomy 237, 264
 expectations of information 45, 49
 package insert 42
 participation groups 49, 80, 181
 rights 45
performance indicators 64, 65, 69, 264
post code 63, 73
practices
 activity analysis 20, 62
 annual report 43
 formulary 190
 group 17, 19, 66
 management 20
 management of change 184
 manager 180, 195
 newsletter 43, 181
 teaching 10, 18
 typical 223
Practitioner, The 26, 28, 33
Prescribers' Journal 28, 35
Prescription Pricing Authority 21, 187, 189
Prestel 101, 107, 122, 194, 214
preventive work 19, 188, 253, 264, 272
problem orientated medical records 7, 8, 228
process tracing 131
profile deprivation 62, 187, 193
protocols 151, 189
Pulse 34

radio
 in health education 109
 phone-ins 56, 111
RAWP 71
record linkage 192, 230, 274, 280
registers
 age–sex 18, 62, 188, 192
 disease *see* 'index, disease'
 E-book 18
Rolleston Committee 4

Royal College of General
    Practitioners
  audit 264
  Birmingham Research Unit
    20
  classification of diseases 18
  Computer Working Party 258
  foundation 5
  influence on GPs' education
    27
  journals monitoring service 31
  Journal of 32, 33
  librarian 29
  publishing activities 30

schools broadcasting 111
screening, developmental 19
shared care 12, 279, *see also*
  card, co-operation
software
  self-assessment 216
  spreadsheet 72, 90
symptom codes 246

tape–slide programmes for
  patients 43
target setting 185, 186
Taylor, S. *Good General
  Practice* 5
Teletext 101, 108, 213
television 109–11
  closed circuit 108, 214
  doctors' antipathy towards
    57, 110, 116
  role in health education 56,
    110
  support services 112

Tonbridge Report 1965 6
transaction of information 225

Update 28, 35

VAMP 73
Viatel 101
video
  interactive 218
  programmes for patients 43
  role in health education 57
Videotex 101, 122, 125, 213
visits, book 187
voluntary organisations 81
  leaflets 44, 54

Walford on summary cards 5
war
  Boer, men unfit for 52
  1914–1918
    dissemination of
      information 53
    effect on medical records
      4
  1939–1945
    genesis of NHS Act 270
    government spending on
      health education 54
Weed, L. — problem orientated
  medical records (q.v.) 7, 228
WONCA journal: *Family
  Practice* 33
World Health Organisation
  Reports
  1954 and 1958 54
  1983 84
World Medicine 35